MEMORY BANK FOR
CRITICAL CAR

EKGs and Cardiac Drugs

3rd Edition

MEMORY BANK FOR
CRITICAL CARE

EKGs and Cardiac Drugs

3rd Edition

Gary W. Ervin, RN
Staff, Kaiser Foundation Hospital
Los Angeles, California

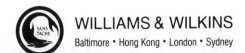

WILLIAMS & WILKINS
Baltimore • Hong Kong • London • Sydney

Editor: Margo C. Neal
Associate Editor: Linda Napora
Copy Editor: Lindsay E. Edmunds
Design: Norman W. Och
Illustration Planning: Wayne Hubbel
Production: Theda Harris

in a review. Printed in the United States of America Library of Congress Cataloging in Publication Data

Ervin, Gary W., 1940§
  Memory bank for critical care : EKGs and cardiac drugs / Gary W. Ervin. — 3rd ed.
      p.   cm.
  Bibliography: p.
  Includes index.
  ISBN 0-683-02820-0
  1. Cardiovascular disease nursing.   2. Intensive care nursing.
3. Electrocardiography.   4. Cardiovascular agents.   I. Title.
  [DNLM: 1. Cardiovascular Agents—nurses' instruction.   2. Critical Care—nurses' instruction.   3. Electrocardiography—nurses' instruction.   4. Heart Diseases—nurses' instruction.   WG 140 E73m]
RC674.E78 1988
616.1028—dc 19
ENLM/DLC
for Library of Congress   88-5453
                                                                            CIP

    90 91 92   10 9 8 7 6 5 4 3

PREFACE

Memory Bank for Critical Care was created to make an immense amount of critical data readily available in a pocket-sized format. It is a ready reference on critical care management that serves two important purposes. First, it facilitates learning and improves comprehension. Second, it fills the need for a concise, on-the-spot reference.

In this, our third edition, we have added both normal and abnormal 12-lead EKG tracings. The pertinent leads for diagnosing such conditions as myocardial infarctions, blocks, and drug effects are provided.

In addition, we have included many new drugs and, where appropriate, have listed the therapeutic levels. We remind the reader that while certain medications are dosed by serum levels, other drugs are regulated by their therapeutic effects. Also, keep in mind that what is therapeutic for one patient may be less than the optimal dosage or toxic in other patients. Additionally, because variations exist among laboratories, keep in mind that the data given in this reference may or may not agree precisely with data from your facility. We suggest you use this information as a guide and not as absolute values. To be certain, check with your laboratory for any variations. We acknowledge that some EKGs may be interpreted differently by different readers. However, the EKGs in this book represent a consensus of the author and the reviewers.

Appreciation is extended to Alden D. Fletcher, MD, and Gary Besinque, PharmD, of Kaiser Foundation Hospital, Los Angeles, for their review of the Cardiology and Pharmacology sections, respectively.

Gary W. Ervin, RN

CONTENTS

SECTION 6: Cardiac Drugs 182

SECTION 7: Terminology 257

SECTION 1

Electrocardiography

TIME MEASUREMENT

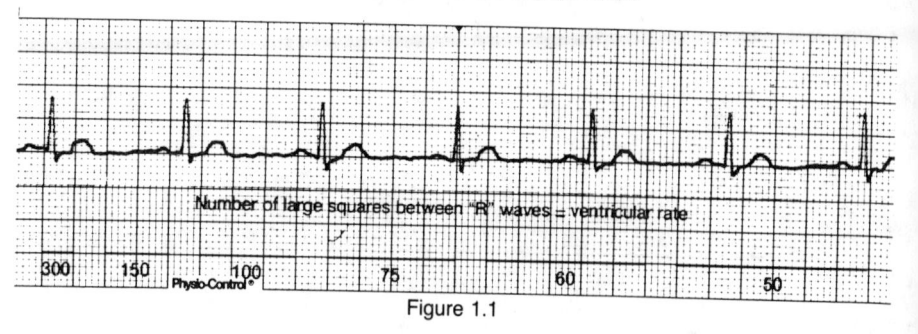

Number of large squares between "R" waves = ventricular rate

300   150   100   75   60   50

Physio-Control®

Figure 1.1

1. Time is measured on the horizontal axis of graph paper.
2. Each minor box = 0.04 second.

3. Each major box = 0.20 second.
4. Five major boxes = 1.0 second = 1 inch of graph paper.
5. 300 major boxes = 1 minute = 60 seconds.
6. Graph paper is marked along the top at 3-second intervals = 3 inches.
7. 6 inches of graph paper = 10 seconds.

RATE DETERMINATION

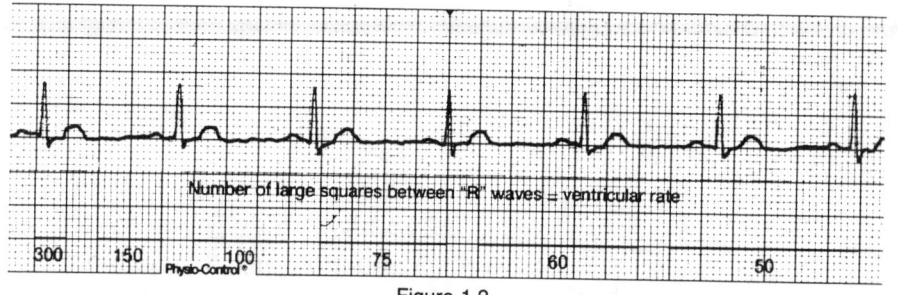

Figure 1.2

1. Count the number of major boxes between two R waves and divide this into 300. For example: 300/4.2 = 73.
2. Or, count the number of R waves in a 6-second strip and multiply by 10.

VOLTAGE MEASUREMENT

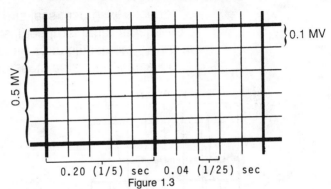

Figure 1.3

1. Voltage is measured on the vertical axis of graph paper.
2. Each minor box = 0.1 mV (when standardized).
3. Each major box = 0.5 mV (when standardized).

P WAVE

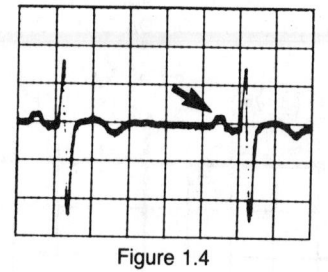

Figure 1.4

1. Represents atrial depolarization.
2. Normally from sinoatrial (SA) node.
3. Sometimes from other atrial sites.
4. Width is less than 0.11 second.

NORMAL P WAVE CONFIGURATIONS

Lead I	Upright
Lead II	Upright
Lead III	Biphasic, flat, or inverted
Lead AVR	Inverted
Lead AVL	Upright, inverted, or biphasic
Lead AVF	Upright

Lead I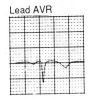

Lead AVR

Lead II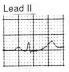

Lead AVL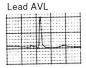

Figure 1.5

Lead III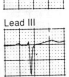

Lead AVF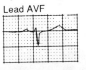

P-R SEGMENT

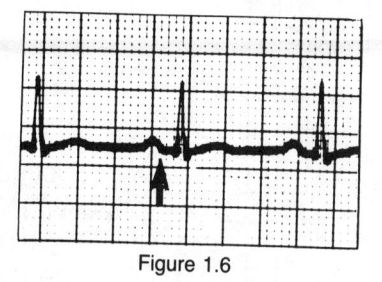

Figure 1.6

1. Distance measured from the end of the P wave to the beginning of the QRS complex.
2. Represents the delay of the sinus impulse through the atrium and atrioventricular (AV) node.

P-R INTERVAL

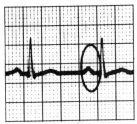

Figure 1.7

1. Distance measured from the beginning of the P wave to the beginning of the QRS complex (P-QRS).
2. Normally 0.12 to 0.20 second.
3. More than 0.20 second is block (conduction defect or chemical).

QRS COMPLEX

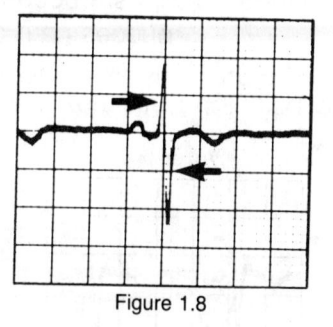

Figure 1.8

1. Represents ventricular depolarization.
2. Width is normally 0.12 second or less (more than 0.12 is block).

Q WAVE

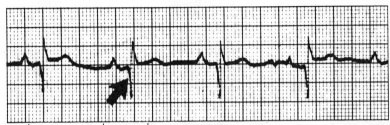

Figure 1.9

1. When the first component of the QRS is a negative deflection, it is called the Q wave.
2. Not always seen in all leads.
3. Normal Q wave duration is 0.03 second or less.
4. Represents septal depolarization in the normal EKG.

R WAVE

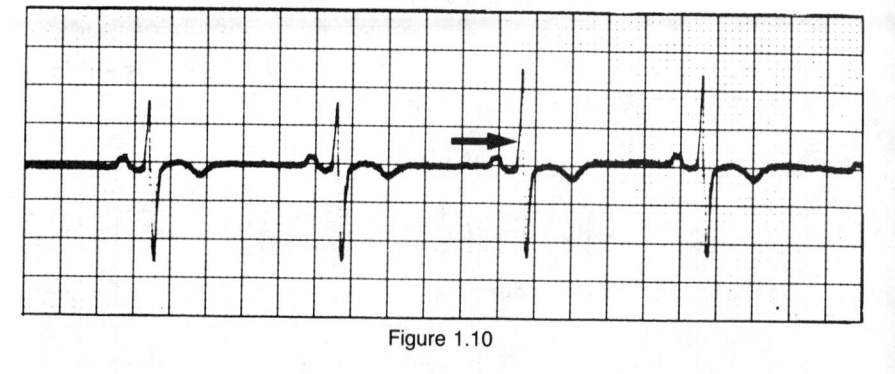

Figure 1.10

The first *positive* deflection of the QRS complex is the R wave.

S WAVE

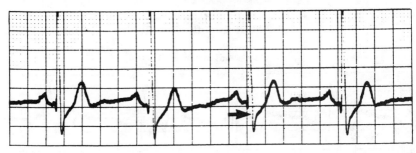

Figure 1.11

The first *negative* deflection after the R wave.

T WAVE

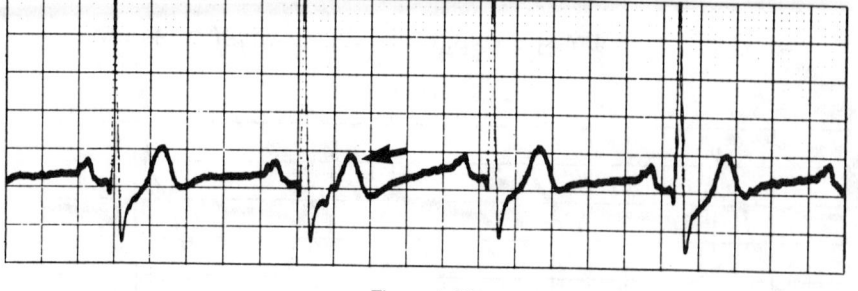

Figure 1.12

Represents repolarization of the ventricles.

NORMAL T-WAVE CONFIGURATIONS

Lead I	Upright
Lead II	Upright
Lead III	Flat, biphasic, or inverted
Lead AVR	Inverted
Lead AVL	Upright, flat, biphasic, or inverted
Lead AVF	Upright, flat, biphasic, or inverted

Figure 1.13

Lead I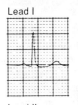
Lead AVR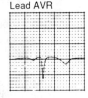

Lead II
Lead AVL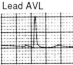

Lead III
Lead AVF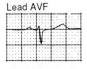

Q-T INTERVAL

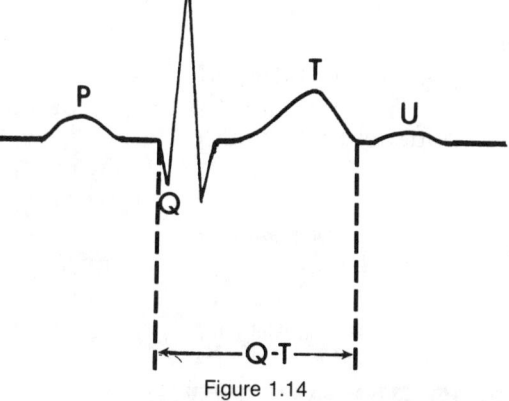
Figure 1.14

1. The time interval required for ventricular depolarization and repolarization.
2. Measured from the beginning of the QRS complex to the end of the T wave.
3. Normal Q-T duration is from 0.30 second to 0.46 second.
4. Q-T interval varies with heart rate (lengthens as heart rate decreases).

S-T SEGMENT

The interval from the end of the QRS to the beginning of the T wave. The normal S-T segment is isoelectric.

Figure 1.15

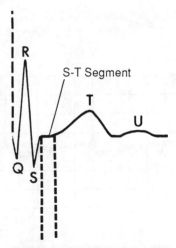

U WAVE

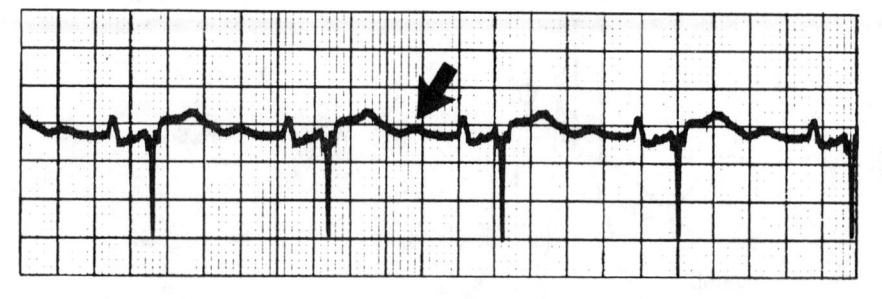

Figure 1.16

1. A minor deflection that sometimes follows the T wave.
2. Genesis uncertain; considered an after potential or result of repolarization of the Perkinje fibers.
3. Indicates hypokalemia if accompanied by a depressed S-T segment in the absence of digitalis preparations.

R¹S¹

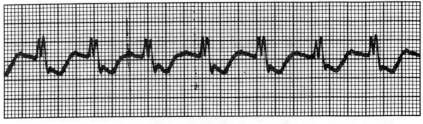

Figure 1.17

1. R¹ is the first positive deflection after the S wave.
2. S¹ is the first negative deflection after the R¹.

SECTION 2
Rhythms and Dysrhythmias

A. SINUS RHYTHMS AND DYSRHYTHMIAS

NORMAL SINUS RHYTHM (NSR)

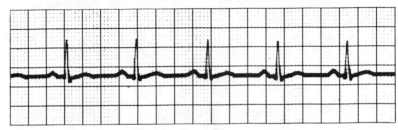

Figure 2.1

1. Rate between 60 and 100.
2. P:QRS = 1:1.
3. Normal intervals and contours.

SINUS DYSRHYTHMIA

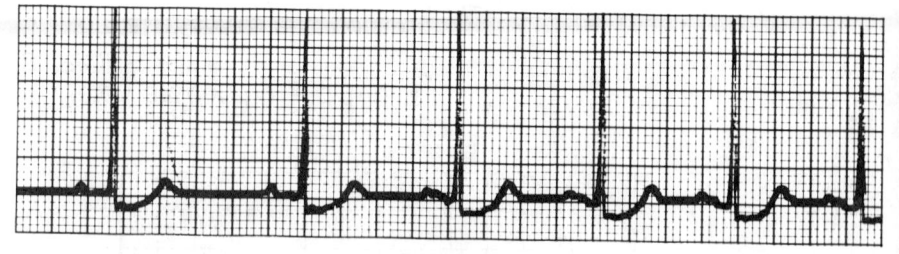

Figure 2.2

1. Rate between 60 and 100.
2. P:QRS = 1:1.
3. Normal intervals and contours.
4. P-P intervals vary more than 0.16 second.

SINUS BRADYCARDIA (SB)

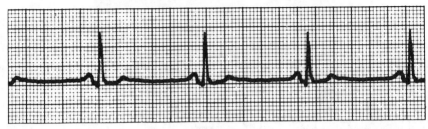

Figure 2.3

1. Rate less than 60.
2. P:QRS = 1:1.
3. Normal intervals and contours.

SINUS TACHYCARDIA (ST)

1. Rate between 100 and 150.
2. P:QRS = 1:1.
3. Normal intervals and contours.

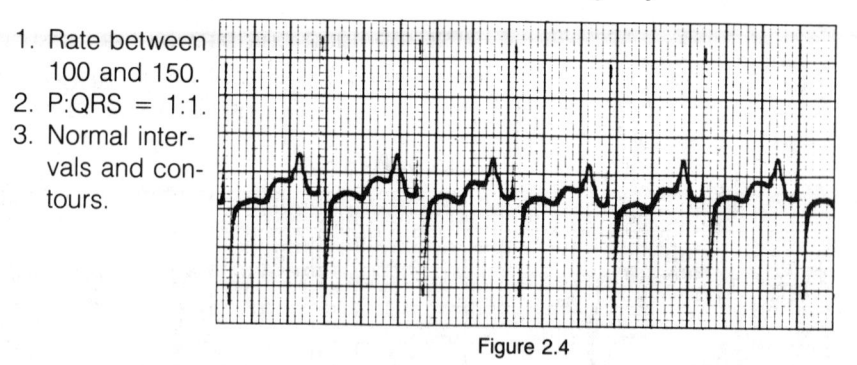

Figure 2.4

SINOATRIAL BLOCK
(SA Block, Sinus Exit Block)

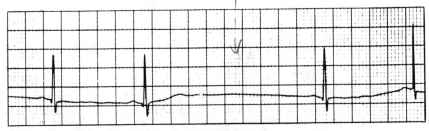

Figure 2.5

1. Absence of normally expected P wave and QRS.
2. Pause = multiple of normal P-P interval.
3. P waves "march through."

SINUS ARREST

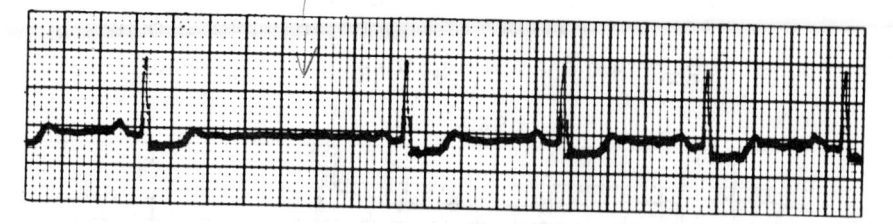

Figure 2.6

1. Pause in cardiac rhythm due to failure of SA node to initiate an impulse.
2. P waves do not "march through."

3. R-R intervals vary because of the pause.
4. Can be life-threatening if prolonged and escape rhythm does not intervene.

B. ATRIAL RHYTHMS AND DYSRHYTHMIAS

PREMATURE ATRIAL CONTRACTION (PAC)

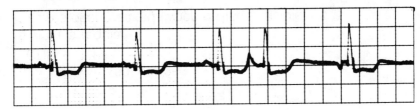

Figure 2.7

1. Premature depolarization of atrial origin.
2. P wave often of different configuration (when visible). May be buried in T wave.
3. P-R interval often different from the dominant P-R.

ATRIAL TACHYCARDIA

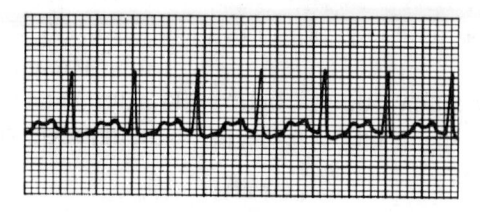

Figure 2.8

1. Rate between 150 and 250.
2. P:QRS = 1:1.
3. Rhythm is regular.
4. P waves often peaked (when distinctly visible).

PAROXYSMAL ATRIAL TACHYCARDIA (PAT)

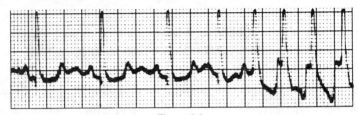

Figure 2.9

1. Rate usually about 150 per minute.
2. Onset and termination abrupt.
3. Usually regular, but can be irregular at the onset and termination of dysrhythmia.
4. Other characteristics as in atrial tachycardia.

ATRIAL FIBRILLATION

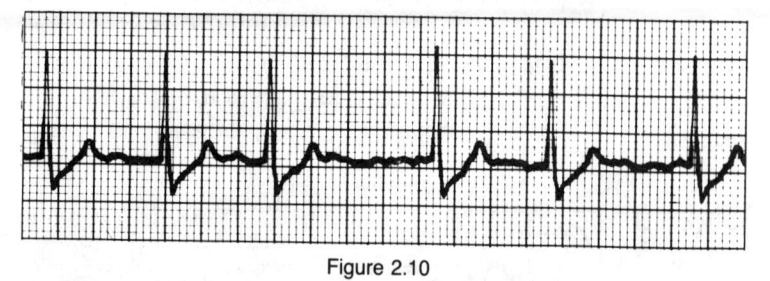

Figure 2.10

1. Atrial rate 350 to 500, and disorganized.
2. Consistent, identifiable P waves are absent.
3. Ventricular response commonly 50 to 200 and irregularly irregular.

ATRIAL FLUTTER

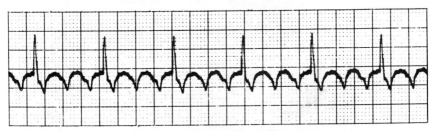

Figure 2.11

1. Rate between 250 and 350 (atrial rate).
2. Ventricular rate usually about 150.
3. Saw-tooth pattern of flutter waves (atrial waves).
4. Atrial rhythm is regular.

WANDERING ATRIAL PACEMAKER
(Multifocal Atrial Impulses)

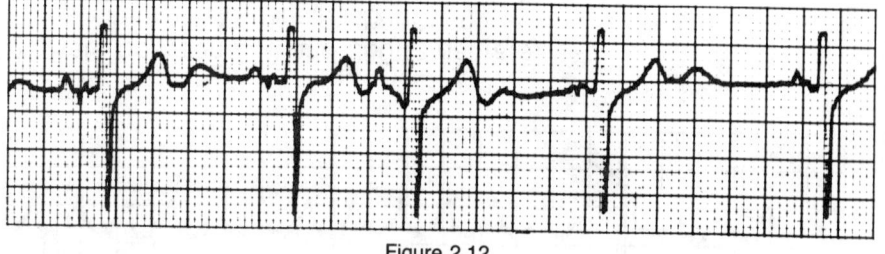

Figure 2.12

1. P waves with at least three different morphologies.
2. P-R intervals vary with the P wave.
3. R-R intervals irregular.

SUPRAVENTRICULAR TACHYCARDIA (SVT)

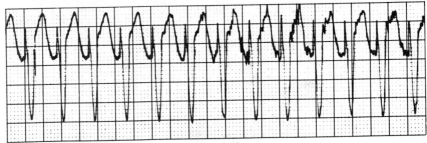

Figure 2.13

1. Ventricular response 150–250. (If the rate is greater than 200, consider Wolff-Parkinson-White syndrome.)
2. P waves obscure in most leads.

3. QRS usually of normal configuration, but aberrant conduction is not unusual.
4. Rhythm regular or irregular.
5. Impulse originates in AV junction or atria.
6. Term SVT is used to label tachydysrhythmias for which origin of impulse formation is not readily identified, except as supraventricular.

C. AV JUNCTIONAL RHYTHMS AND DYSRHYTHMIAS

JUNCTIONAL RHYTHM

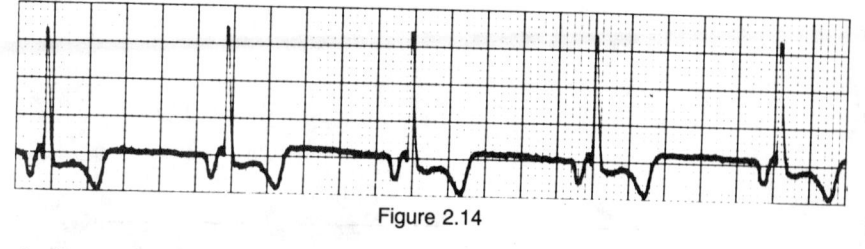

Figure 2.14

1. Rate between 35 and 60.
2. Junctional P wave may precede, be buried in, or follow the QRS.
3. When seen, the junctional P wave is inverted (retrograde depolarization) and the P-R interval is less than 0.12 second.
4. Rhythm is usually regular.

ACCELERATED JUNCTIONAL RHYTHM

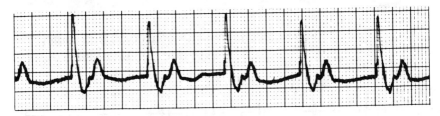

Figure 2.15

1. Rate between 60 and 100.
2. Other characteristics as in junctional rhythm.

JUNCTIONAL TACHYCARDIA

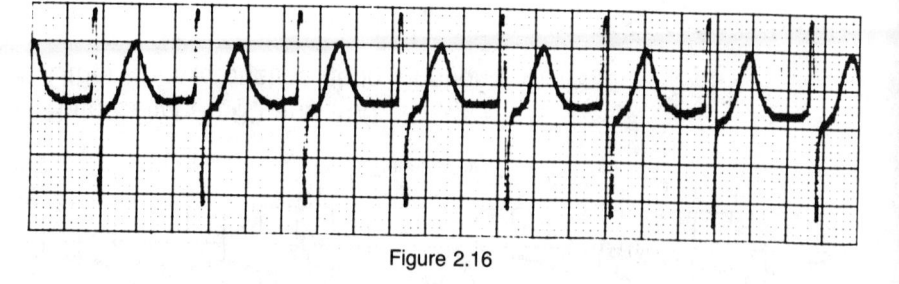

Figure 2.16

1. Rate between 100 and 200.
2. Other characteristics as in junctional rhythm.

PREMATURE JUNCTIONAL CONTRACTION (PJC)

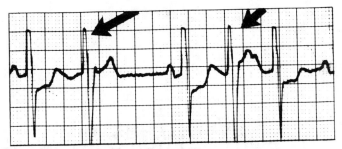

Figure 2.17

1. Premature depolarization.
2. Atrioventricular (AV) junctional origin.
3. Other characteristics as in junctional rhythm.

D. VENTRICULAR RHYTHMS AND DYSRHYTHMIAS

IDIOVENTRICULAR RHYTHM

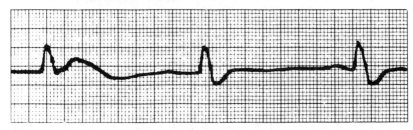

Figure 2.18

1. Ventricular rate between 20 and 40.
2. QRS complex 0.12 second or wider.
3. Rhythm is regular.

propapenone

ACCELERATED IDIOVENTRICULAR RHYTHM

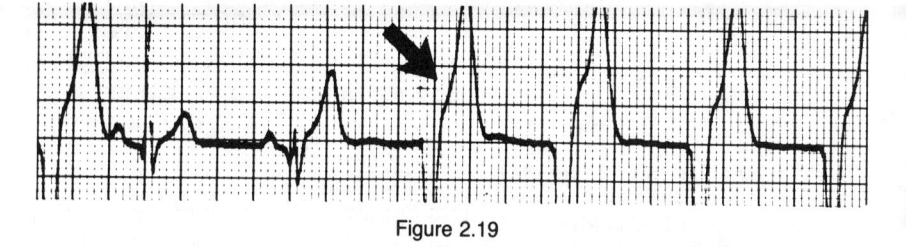

Figure 2.19

1. Rate between 40 and 100.
2. QRS 0.12 second or wider.
3. Rhythm is regular.
4. Runs of accelerated ventricular rhythm usually preceded and followed by fusion beats.

PREMATURE VENTRICULAR CONTRACTIONS
(PVCs)

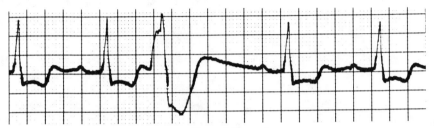

Figure 2.20

1. Premature contractions of ventricular origin.
2. Complex is wide (0.12 second or more), usually followed by a compensatory pause (either fully or partially compensatory).

3. T wave usually large and opposite main deflection.
4. May fuse with supraventricular focus.
5. Unifocal PVCs couple.
6. May be interpolated (does not interfere with regular sinus rhythm).

MULTIFOCAL PVCs

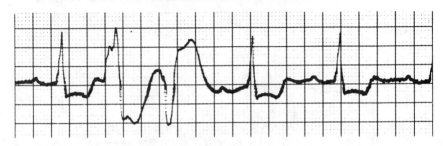

Figure 2.21

1. PVCs from different points of focus.
2. PVCs with different configurations.
3. Coupling intervals are different.

INTERPOLATED PVCs

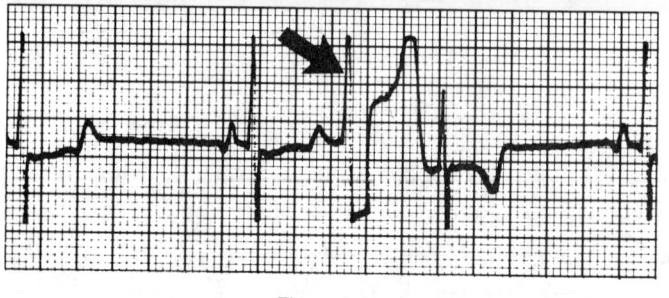

Figure 2.22

1. Premature beat of ventricular origin that does not disturb the sinus rhythm.
2. Complex wide (0.12 second or more).

3. The following P wave is on time, but may conduct with a prolonged P-R interval.
4. No compensatory pause.

BIGEMINAL RHYTHM

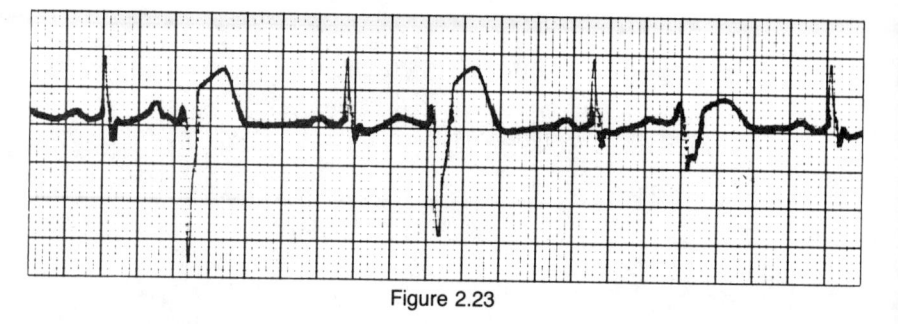

Figure 2.23

Rhythm that consists of pairs of beats, as with a sinus beat followed by an ectopic beat (PAC, PJC, or PVC) in a 1:1 ratio.

TRIGEMINAL RHYTHM

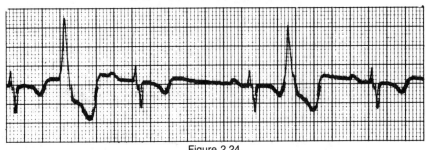

Figure 2.24

Trios of beats, as with two sinus beats followed by an ectopic beat (PAC, PJC, or PVC) in a 2:1 ratio.

PRELETHAL (COMPLEX) VENTRICULAR DYSRHYTHMIAS

1. R on T phenomena.
2. More than six PVCs per minute.
3. Bigeminal PVCs.
4. Multifocal PVCs.
5. Back to back PVCs.
6. Ventricular tachycardia.

VENTRICULAR TACHYCARDIA (V-Tach)

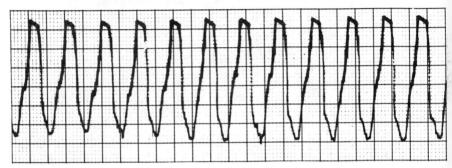

Figure 2.25

1. Three or more successive ventricular beats with a rate 100-200.
2. QRS wider than 0.12 second.
3. Rhythm is essentially regular.
4. Life-threatening dysrhythmia.

TORSADES DE POINTES
(VENTRICULAR FLUTTER)

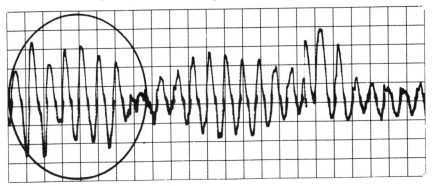

Figure 2.26

1. Rate 150-300.
2. A rapid, regular, ventricular tachycardia.
3. QRSs resemble sine waves.

VENTRICULAR FIBRILLATION (V-Fib)

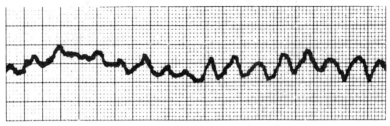

Figure 2.27

1. Rhythm is grossly irregular in contour and amplitude.
2. Nondistinct QRS complexes.
3. Lethal dysrhythmia.

AGONAL RHYTHM

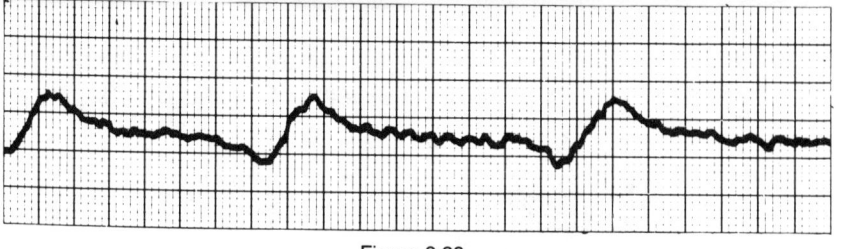

Figure 2.28

1. Fine ventricular fibrillation.
2. Usually precedes asystole.

ASYSTOLE

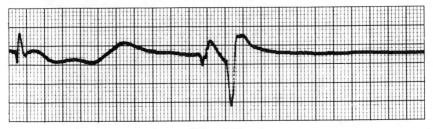

Figure 2.29

1. Ventricular standstill
2. "Straight line" on monitor.

E. CONDUCTION ANOMALIES

AV BLOCK, 1st DEGREE

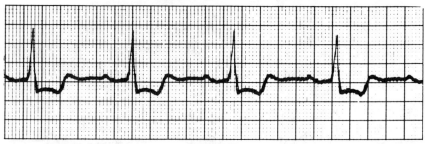

Figure 2.30

1. P-R interval more than 0.20 second.
2. Rhythm remains regular.

AV BLOCK, 2nd DEGREE
(Mobitz Type I—Wenckebach Phenomenon)

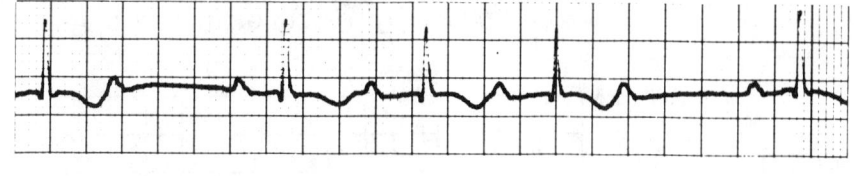

Figure 2.31

1. 2nd-degree AV block.
2. P waves remain regular.
3. Not all atrial impulses are conducted.

4. Progressive lengthening of P-R interval until one P wave is not conducted.
5. Progressive shortening of R-R interval until one P wave is not conducted.

AV BLOCK, 2nd DEGREE
(Mobitz Type II)

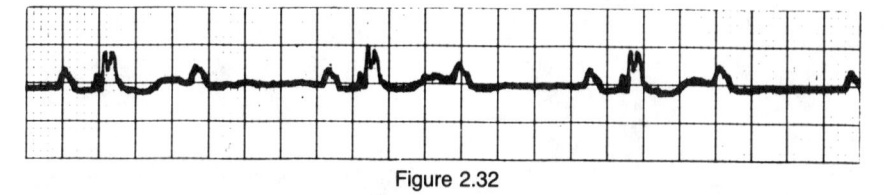

Figure 2.32

1. Constant atrial rate, 60-100.
2. More P waves than QRS complexes.
3. Ventricular response commonly in 2:1 or 3:1 configuration, but may vary.
4. No change in the P-R intervals of conducted P waves.

AV BLOCK, 3rd DEGREE
(Complete AV Block)

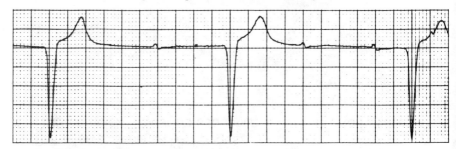

Figure 2.33

1. No conduction of atrial impulses.
2. Atria and ventricles beat independently, and P:QRS have no sequential relationship.
3. Regular atrial and ventricular rates.
4. P-R interval continually changes.
5. QRS complexes bear no sequential relationship to P waves.

odchylenie

ABERRANT VENTRICULAR CONDUCTION
(AVC)

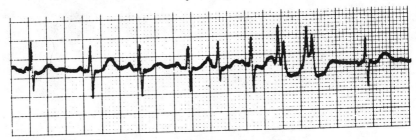

Figure 2.34

1. Aberrant ventricular conduction of premature supraventricular impulse.

2. Most AVCs look like right bundle branch block (RSR^1) in V$_1$ and MCL$_1$.
3. Coupling is not fixed.
4. AVCs tend to be either isolated or in runs rather than in patterns (bigeminy, trigeminy).

ASHMAN PHENOMENON

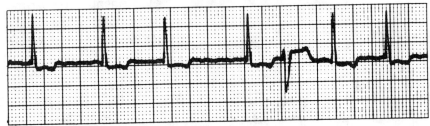

Figure 2.35

1. A prolonged R-R interval is followed by a short R-R interval where the QRS conducts aberrantly.
2. Commonly seen in atrial fibrillation.

FUSION BEATS

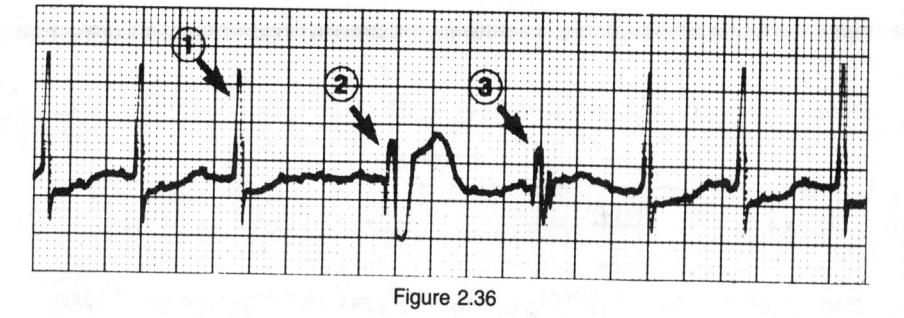

Figure 2.36

Arrow #1 = intrinsic QRS
Arrow #2 = paced QRS
Arrow #3 = fused QRS

1. Simultaneous depolarization of heart by two foci.
2. QRS configuration different from intrinsic and ectopic (or paced) configurations.

PARASYSTOLE

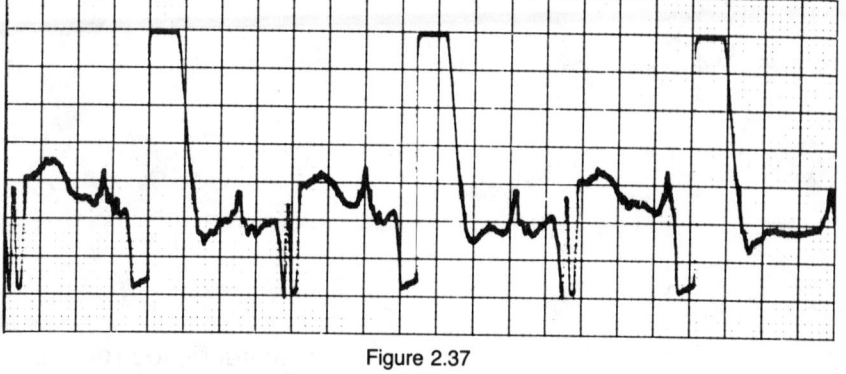

Figure 2.37

1. Coupling interval varies.
2. Ectopic that fires at a fixed rate.
3. Ectopic focus is "protected," and dominant rhythm does not depolarize ectopic site.
4. Intervals between parasystoles reduce to a common denominator.
5. Fusion beats are common.
6. May be atrial, junctional, or ventricular in origin.
7. Rarely caused by digitalis toxicity.

PRE-EXCITATION SYNDROME CHARACTERISTICS

1. Pre-excitation = abnormally early activation of the ventricles via accessory pathways that bypass the AV node.
2. With normal P wave configuration, the P-R interval is short (usually 0.12 second or less).
3. Propensity to rapid, aberrant SVTs that mimic V-tach (rates of 250–300 are not uncommon) and that may degenerate into V-fib and sudden death.
4. Pre-excitation syndrome includes Wolff-Parkinson-White (type A and type B) and Lown-Ganong-Levine syndromes.

LOWN-GANONG-LEVINE (LGL)

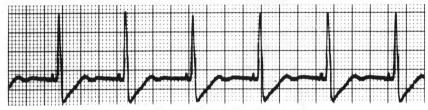

Figure 2.38

1. Short P-R interval with narrow QRS (unless bundle branch block exists).
2. Accessory pathway from atrium to junction of AV node and His bundle.
3. Incidence about 70% in females with a propensity to hypertension and rapid, aberrant SVTs.

WOLFF-PARKINSON-WHITE (WPW)

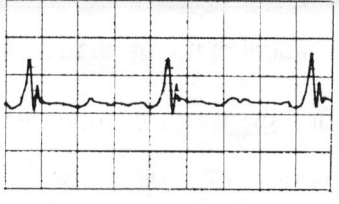

Figure 2.39

1. Short P-R interval with prolonged QRS.
2. Incidence about 70% in males.
3. Type A = accessory pathway between left atrium and left ventricle. Look for Delta wave (slurred R wave) in V_1 and V_2.

4. Type B = accessory pathway between right atrium and right ventricle. Look for a large Q wave in V_1 and V_2. (Above strip is WPW, type A.)

F. PACEMAKERS

GENERAL COMMENTS

1. A pacemaker is a device that provides electrical impulses that initiate and/or maintain a cardiac rhythm.
2. The demand pacemaker provides a rhythm when the intrinsic rhythm fails.
3. Pacing units can be either temporary or permanent.
4. Indications for pacers include sick sinus syndrome, symptomatic bradycardia, complete heart block, and second-degree heart block (Mobitz type II).

PACEMAKER SPIKE

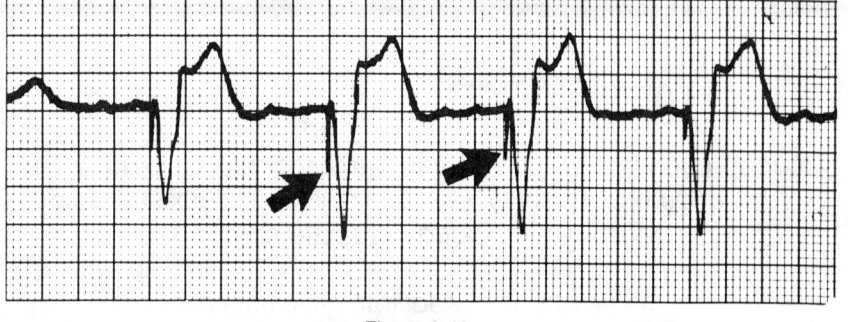

Figure 2.40

1. The pacemaker spike represents the electrical impulse and is the pacemaker inscription or artifact.
2. The pacemaker spike is represented by a vertical line on the graph paper.

ATRIAL PACEMAKER

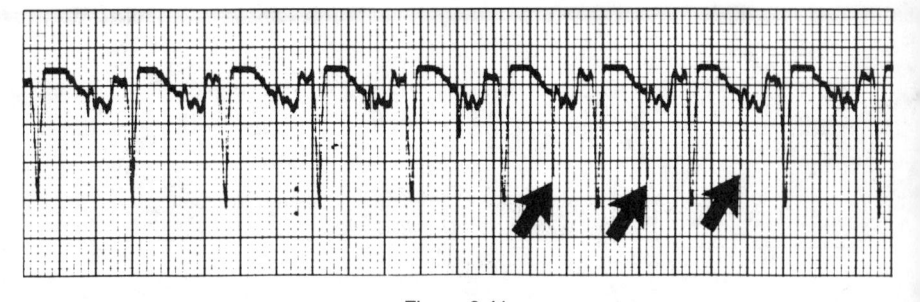

Figure 2.41

1. Indicated when sinoatrial (SA) node is diseased or damaged, but the AV conduction system remains intact.

2. In effect, the atrial pacemaker replaces the SA impulse and initiates atrial contraction.
3. The atria contract and pump blood to the ventricles (atrial kick); can add from 5–25% to cardiac output over a ventricular pacemaker.
4. The QRS appearance is the same as the intrinsic complexes.

VENTRICULAR DEMAND PACEMAKER

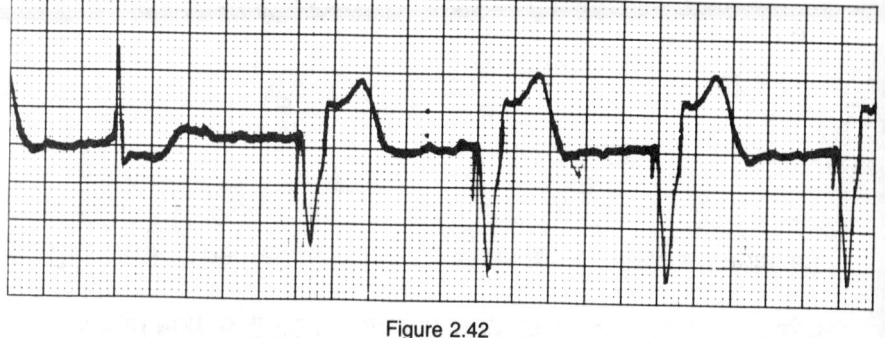

Figure 2.42

1. Indicated in instances of complete heart block.
2. Ventricular filling probably not as complete as with AV synchronous rhythms.
3. QRS complexes appear similar to right-sided PVCs. (In the above strip, the intrinsic beat is followed by a ventricular-paced, escape rhythm.)

ATRIAL-VENTRICULAR SEQUENTIAL PACEMAKER

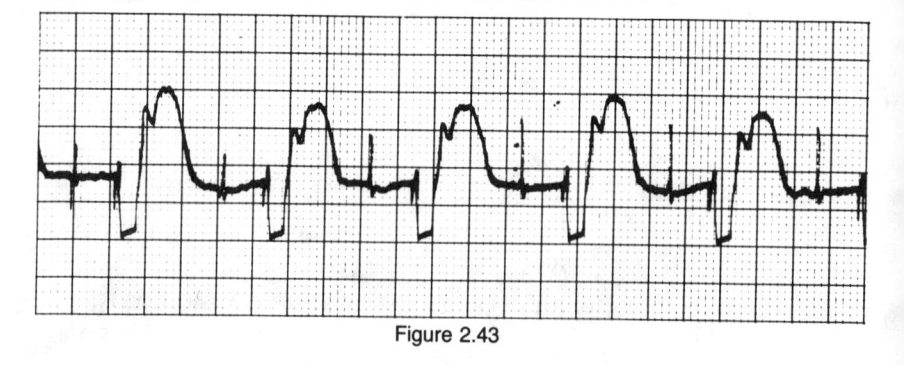

Figure 2.43

1. Provides atrial and ventricular pacing in sequence.
2. Atrial contraction assures more complete ventricular filling than the ventricular demand pacing unit.

PACEMAKER MALFUNCTIONS

1. Failure to capture.
2. Failure to sense.
3. Runaway pacemaker.

FAILURE TO CAPTURE

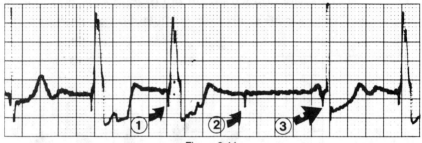

Figure 2.44

This is the description used when the pacemaker impulse fails to cause ventricular contraction (fails to "capture" the ventricles).

FAILURE TO SENSE

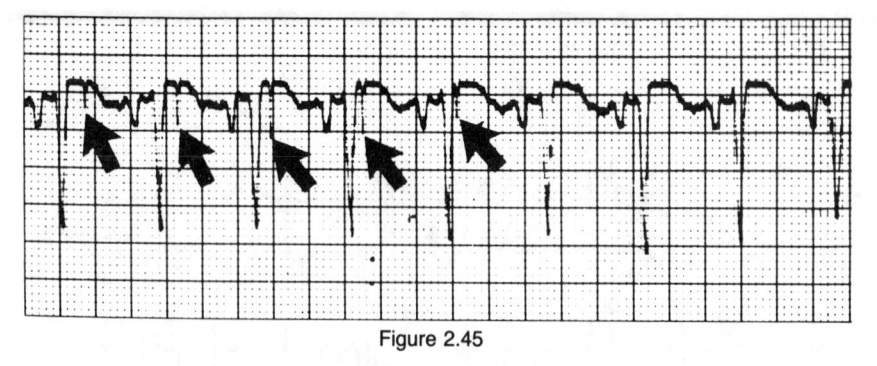

Figure 2.45

This is when the demand pacemaker does not detect an intrinsic beat and fires prior to the preset escape interval.

SECTION 3
12-Lead EKG

A. LEADS

FRONTAL LEADS

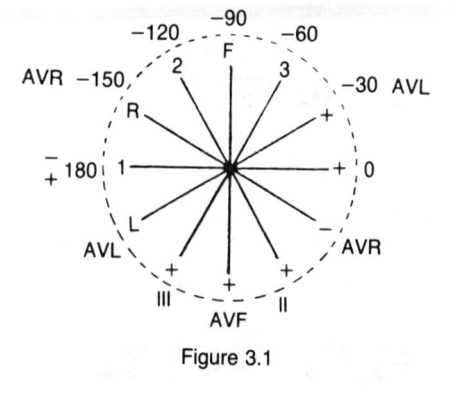

Figure 3.1

Lead		Vector	Strongest Normal Deflection
I	(left lead)	0 degrees	+
II	(inferior lead)	+60 degrees	strong +
III	(inferior lead)	+120 degrees	weak +
AVR	(right lead)	−150 degrees	strong -
AVL	(left lead)	−30 degrees	equaphasic
AVF	(inferior lead)	+90 degrees	strong +

HORIZONTAL LEADS

Lead	Focus
V₁	Septal
V₂–V₄	Anterior
V₅, V₆, I, AVL	Lateral

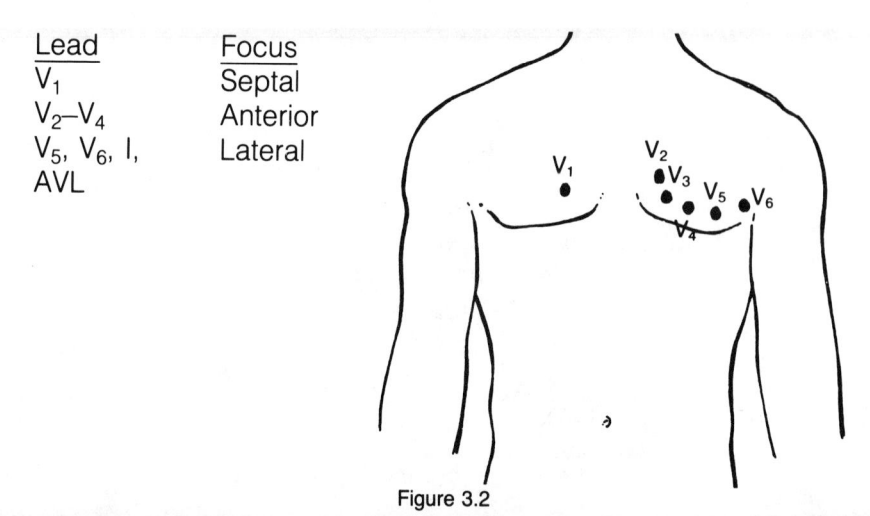

Figure 3.2

LEFT HEART LEADS

I, AVL, V_5, and V_6

PERPENDICULAR LEADS

Lead		Perpendicular To
I	(0 degrees)	AVF (+90 degrees)
II	(+60 degrees)	AVL (−30 degrees)
III	(+120 degrees)	AVR (−150 degrees)

(see Figure 3.1)

RIGHT HEART LEADS

V_1, V_2, and AVR

STANDARD LIMB LEADS

Lead I   Right Arm (−)
              to Left Arm (+)

Lead II   Right Arm (−)
              to Left Leg (+)

Lead III   Left Arm (−)
              to Left Leg (+)

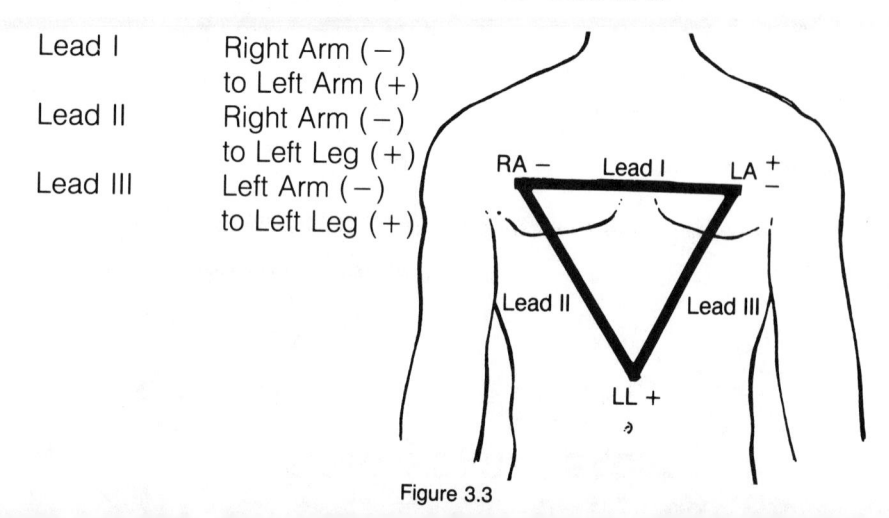

Figure 3.3

B. BUNDLE BRANCH CONDUCTION, BLOCKS, AND ANOMALIES

BUNDLE BRANCH CONDUCTION

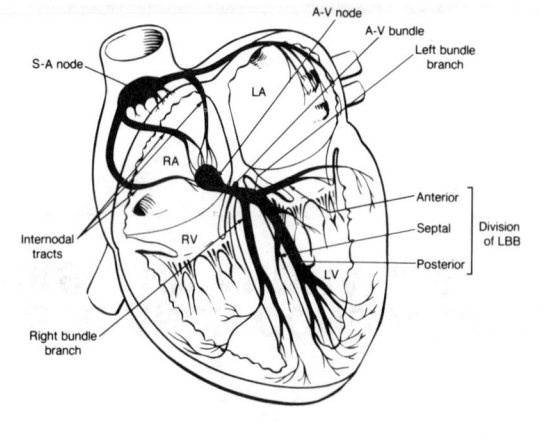

Figure 3.4

1. Right bundle innervates right ventricle.
2. Left posterior fascicle innervates posterior and inferior left ventricular wall.
3. Left anterior fascicle innervates anterior and superior left ventricular wall.

DETERMINATION OF BLOCKS

1. Limb leads determine hemiblocks.
2. Chest leads determine bundle branch blocks.

LEFT ANTERIOR HEMIBLOCK (LAH)
or LEFT ANTERIOR FASCICULAR BLOCK

1. Lead II, small R, deep S
2. Left axis deviation (−30° or greater).

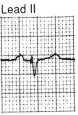

Lead II

Figure 3.5

LEFT POSTERIOR HEMIBLOCK (LPH)
or LEFT POSTERIOR FASCICULAR BLOCK

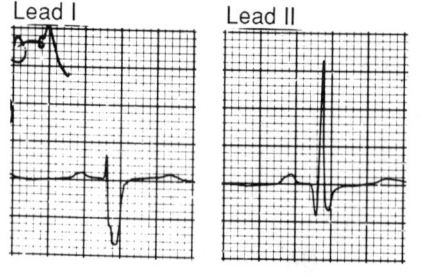

Figure 3.6

1. Lead I, small R, deep and wide S, negative QRS (RS).
2. Leads II and III, small Q, tall R, positive QRS.
3. Right axis deviation.

LEFT COMPLETE BUNDLE BRANCH BLOCK (LBBB)

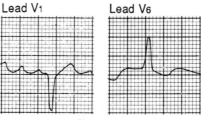

Figure 3.7

1. Small or absent R waves in leads V_1 through V_3 with wide S waves.
2. Tall and prolonged R waves in leads V_5 and V_6.
3. T wave in opposite direction to the major QRS deflection.

RIGHT COMPLETE BUNDLE BRANCH BLOCK (RBBB)

Lead V₁

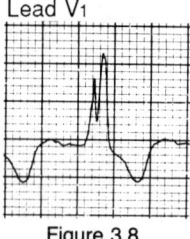

Figure 3.8

1. Lead V_1, late positive vector (RSR[1]), QRS duration longer than 0.12 second.
2. Wide S in leads I, V_5, and V_6.

AXIS DEVIATION

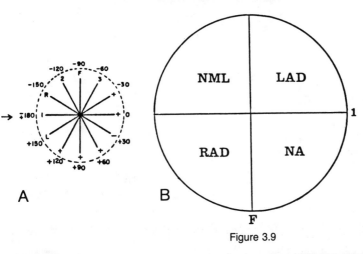

Figure B

LAD = Left Axis
    Deviation
NA = Normal Axis
RAD = Right Axis
    Deviation
NML = No Man's
    Land

A

B

Figure 3.9

1. Normal axis (NA) from +90 degrees to −30 degrees.
2. Left axis deviation (LAD) from −30 to −90 degrees.
3. Right axis deviation (RAD) from +90 to −90 degrees.
4. NML = no man's land.

LEFT AXIS DEVIATION

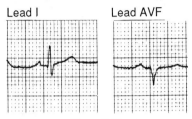

Figure 3.10

1. Mean QRS vector between -30 and -90 degrees.
2. Positive QRS in lead I and negative QRS in lead AVF.

3. Possible etiologies include normal variation, left anterior hemiblock, LBBB, WPW syndrome, emphysema, hyperkalemia, left ventricular enlargement, and congenital lesions.

RIGHT AXIS DEVIATION

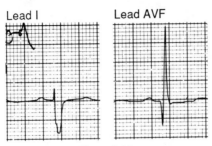

Figure 3.11

1. Mean QRS vector between +110 to −90 degrees (negative QRS in lead I).

2. Possible etiologies include normal variation, right ventricular enlargement, RBBB, left posterior hemiblock, dextrocardia, WPW syndrome, and chronic destructive lung disease.

C. ENLARGEMENT

LEFT ATRIAL ENLARGEMENT

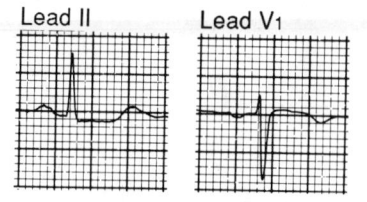

Figure 3.12

1. P wave duration longer than 0.11 second.
2. P wave notched and slurred in leads I and II.
3. Biphasic P waves with wide, deep terminal components in leads V_1 and V_2.

LEFT VENTRICULAR ENLARGEMENT

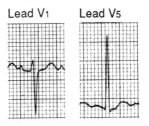

Lead V₁ Lead V₅

Figure 3.13

1. Tall R waves in leads V_5, V_6, I, and AVL.
2. Deep S in leads V_1 and V_2.
3. S-T depression and T wave inversion in leads I, AVL, V_5, and V_6.

RIGHT ATRIAL ENLARGEMENT

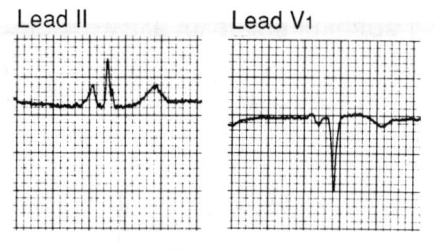

Figure 3.14

1. Tall, peaked P waves in leads II, III, AVF (P pulmonale).
2. Biphasic P waves in leads V_1 and V_2.
3. Normal P wave duration (less than 0.11 second).

RIGHT VENTRICULAR ENLARGEMENT

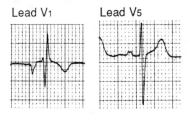

Lead V$_1$ Lead V$_5$

Figure 3.15

1. Tall R in leads V$_1$ and V$_2$.
2. Deep S in leads V$_5$ and V$_6$.
3. Right axis deviation (most useful criterion).

4. Right bundle branch block.
5. Depressed S-T, inverted T waves in leads V_1 and V_2, and leads II, III, AVF.

D. EKG CHANGES

INJURY (ACUTE)

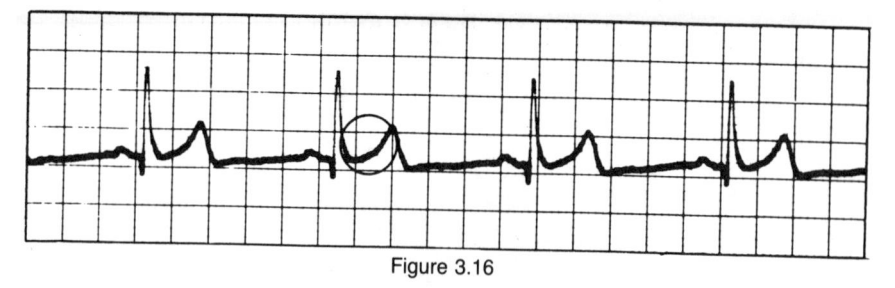

Figure 3.16

1. Damage to myocardium, but not necrosis.
2. Elevated S-T segments in leads that look directly at injured area.

ISCHEMIA

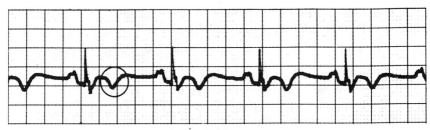

Figure 3.17

1. Myocardial damage that is not yet irreversible.
2. T wave inverted in leads that look directly at ischemic area.
3. With S-T straightening or coving, suspect ischemia.

NECROSIS

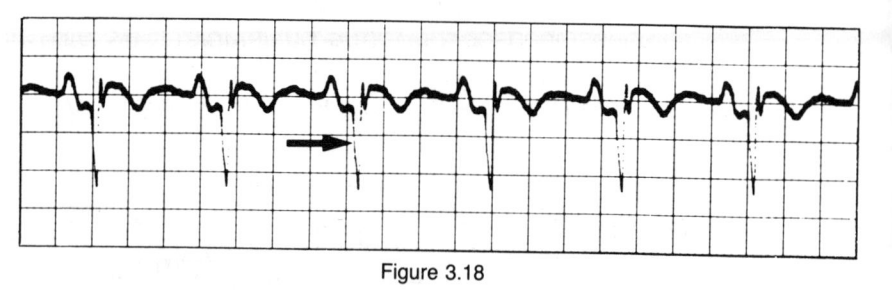

Figure 3.18

1. Death of cells and tissue.
2. Large Q waves in leads that look directly at necrotic area (pathologic Q waves).

PATHOLOGIC Q WAVES

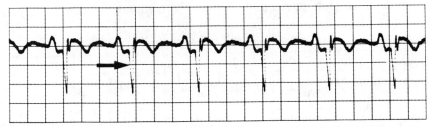

Figure 3.19

1. Width is greater than 0.03 second.
2. Depth is greater than 25% of R wave.

STRAIN PATTERN
Strain Pattern M(Secondary ST-T Changes)

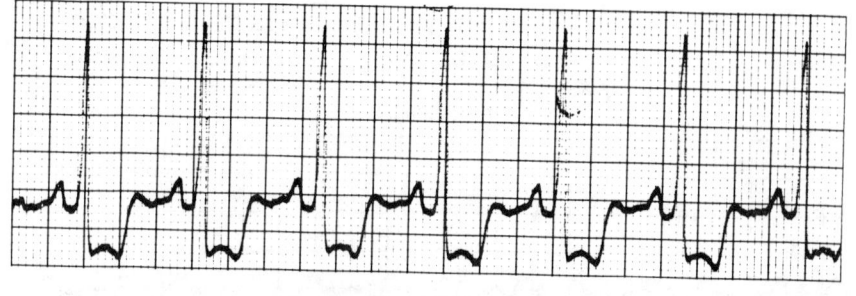

Figure 3.20

1. Characterized by depressed S-T segments and inverted T waves.

2. Develops in patients with long-standing left ventricular enlargement.
3. Strain pattern increases when left ventricular failure and dilatation occur.
4. Mechanism of "strain pattern" not understood.

E. MYOCARDIAL INFARCTION (MI)

ANTERIOR MI

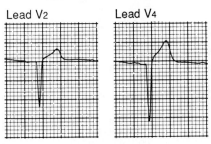

Figure 3.21

Pathologic Q waves in leads V_2–V_4.

ANTEROLATERAL MI

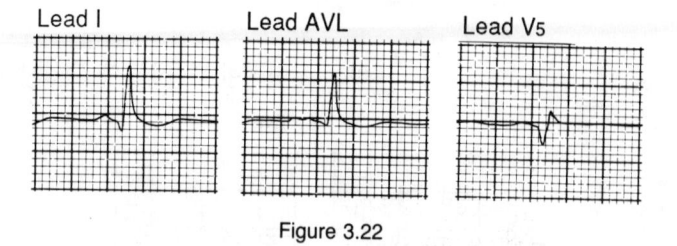

Figure 3.22

Pathologic Q waves in leads I, AVL, and V_4–V_6.

ANTEROSEPTAL MI

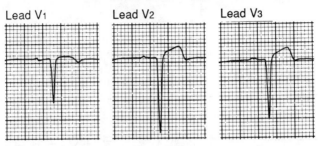

Figure 3.23

Pathologic Q waves in leads V_1–V_3.

EXTENSIVE ANTEROLATERAL MI

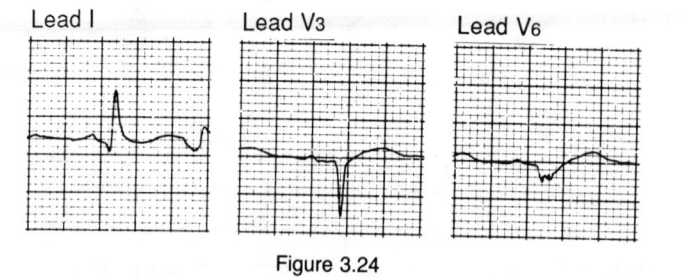

Figure 3.24

Pathologic Q waves in leads I, AVL, and V₁–V₆.

INFERIOR MI

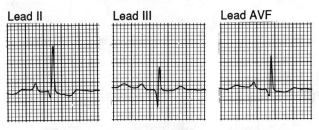

Figure 3.25

Pathologic Q waves in leads II, III, and AVF.

POSTERIOR MI

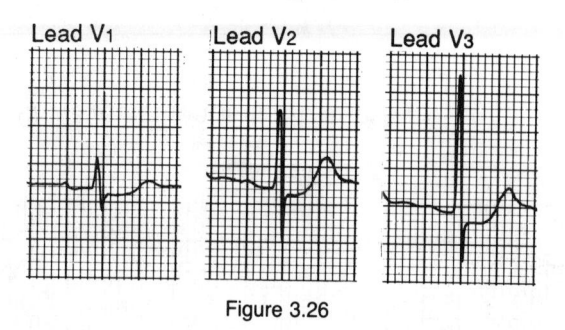

Figure 3.26

1. Tall R wave in V_1–V_3.
2. S-T depression.
3. T wave upright.

SUBENDOCARDIAL MI (Non-Q Wave)

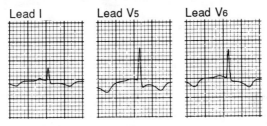

Figure 3.27

1. No pathologic Q waves.
2. Some loss of R waves.
3. Depressed S-T segment.
4. Deep symmetrical T-wave inversion.

F. DRUG AND ELECTROLYTE IMBALANCE EFFECTS

DIGITALIS EFFECT

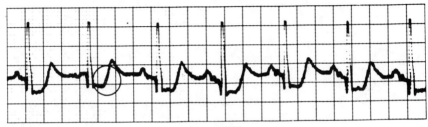

Figure 3.28

1. S-T depression may cover T wave in leads where QRS is positive.
2. Short Q-T interval (similar to hypercalcemia).

DIGITALIS TOXICITY

1. Depressed S-T segment in leads with negative QRS complexes.
2. P-R prolongation (1st-degree block).
3. Mobitz II block with increased atrial activity (PAT with block).
4. Multifocal PVCs.
5. Any atrioventricular (AV) block and sinoatrial (SA) block.
6. Any dysrhythmia except atrial fibrillation with a rapid ventricular response.

HYPERCALCEMIA

1. Q-T interval shortens.
2. S-T segment shortens and may be absent.
3. When advanced, ventricular dysrhythmias.
4. Increased heart tonicity.
5. Systolic arrest (tight arrest).
6. From rapid i.v. infusion: V-Fib and sudden death, especially when patient is receiving digitalis preparations.

Lead V2

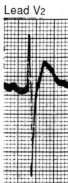

Figure 3.29

HYPOCALCEMIA

1. Lengthened Q-T interval.
2. Lowering and inversion of T wave.
3. Lenthening of S-T segment.
4. Decreased heart tonicity.
5. "Flabby" arrest, although the EKG monitor may look normal.

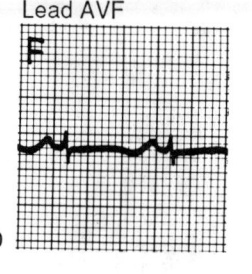

Lead AVF

Figure 3.30

HYPERKALEMIA

Lead II

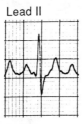

Figure 3.31

1. Peaked T waves, flattened P waves in leads V_2–V_4.
2. AV block.
3. Widened QRS (intraventricular block) to ventricular fibrillation.

HYPOKALEMIA

1. U wave, notched T wave, prolonged Q-T interval.
2. T wave may flatten and invert.
3. S-T segment becomes depressed (as seen in digitalis effect).
4. Peaked P waves in leads II, III, and AVF (pseudo P pulmonale).

Lead V6

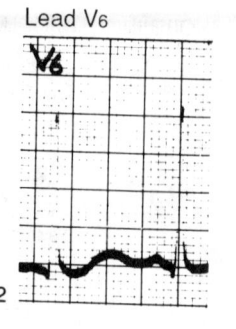

Figure 3.32

QUINIDINE EFFECT

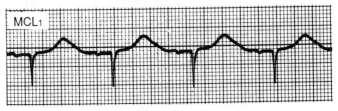

Figure 3.33

1. Widened Q-T interval (similar to hypocalcemia).
2. Widened P waves.
3. Everything slows and spreads out.
4. SA rate slows.

5. Widened QRS (greater than 25% = toxicity).
6. Can cause ventricular dysrhythmias at toxic levels, reentry phenomenon.

SECTION 4

Physical Assessment

A. HEART SOUNDS

CHARACTERISTICS OF HEART SOUNDS

1. Intensity (amplitude).
2. Pitch (high, medium, low frequency).
3. Duration (length of sound).
4. Timbre (quality dependent upon overtones).

LOCATION OF HEART SOUNDS

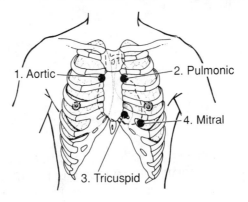

Figure 4.1

1. Aortic heard at 2nd right interspace and left sternal border.
2. Pulmonic heard at 2nd left interspace.
3. Tricuspid heard best at lower left sternal border.
4. Mitral heard at 5th left interspace, midclavicular line (in the normal heart). Corresponds to the apex of the heart.

FIRST HEART SOUND (S₁)

1. Represents onset of systole.
2. Closure of mitral and tricuspid valves.
3. Heard best at apex and lower left sternal border.
4. Corresponds with ventricular depolarization.

SECOND HEART SOUND (S₂)

1. Represents onset of diastole.
2. Closure of aortic and pulmonic valves.
3. Heard best at aortic and pulmonic sites.
4. Splitting of S₂ heard best at pulmonic area with inspiration.
5. Split S₂ at apex suggestive of increased pulmonic relaxation.

THIRD HEART SOUND (S₃)

1. Represents pathology in the adult.
2. Caused by rapid filling against a nonpliable ventricular wall.
3. Heard early in diastole after closure of semilunar valves.
4. Indicates left ventricular failure (an early sign) and/or right failure.
5. Cadence similar to the word "Kentucky."
6. Heard best with bell of stethoscope at lower left sternal border for right-sided failure and at apex for left-sided failure.
7. Ventricular gallop rhythm is exaggerated S₃.

FOURTH HEART SOUND (S₄)

1. Results from atrial contractions against decreased ventricular compliance.
2. Best heard at apex (left ventricle) and lower end of the sternum (right ventricle).
3. Atrial gallop rhythm.
4. Suspect atrioventricular (AV) block, acute MI, congestive heart failure (CHF), and hypertension.
5. Cadence similar to the word "Tennessee."
6. Lower-pitched sound heard best with bell of stethoscope.

SUMMATION GALLOP

1. Found in adults with severe heart disease and tachycardia.
2. Summation of S_3 and S_4.

MURMURS

1. In an adult, a murmur is an abnormal heart sound.
2. Murmurs are vibrations that are audible and caused by turbulent blood flow.
3. Intensity refers to the relative loudness of the murmur and is graded from 1 through 6 (softest through loudest).
4. Quality refers to the tone (musical, blowing, harsh, rumbling).
5. Pitch may be high, medium, or low.
6. Location is determined by where the murmur is most audible.
7. Midsystolic clicks (associated with mitral or tricuspid valve prolapse) may accompany murmurs.
8. Time of murmur refers to when it occurs in the cardiac cycle (systolic or diastolic).

SYSTOLIC MURMUR

1. Most common of all murmurs.
2. Occurs during ventricular contraction (between S_1 and S_2) simultaneously with pulse.
3. Includes midsystolic and holosystolic murmurs.
4. Results from turbulent blood flow through damaged valves, valvular regurgitation, arteriovenous communication, high output states, and aortic stenosis.

MIDSYSTOLIC MURMUR

1. Ejection murmur.
2. Onset after S_1, which crescendos in midsystole and terminates prior to S_2.
3. Murmur of aortic and pulmonic stenosis, high output, and aortic sclerosis.
4. Usually harsh or musical.
5. Heard best over the affected valve.

HOLOSYSTOLIC MURMUR

1. Regurgitant murmur.
2. Duration is throughout systole.
3. Quality may be blowing, musical, or harsh.
4. Heard best over affected area.
5. Causes include chronic tricuspid and mitral insufficiency and ventricular septal defects.

DIASTOLIC MURMUR

1. Onset is after pulse is felt, between S_2 and S_1.
2. Murmur of regurgitation of aortic and pulmonic valves.
3. Usually high pitched, blowing, and decrescendo.
4. Tricuspid stenosis best heard over tricuspid site.
5. Mitral stenosis is best heard at apex as low pitched and frequently preceded by an opening snap.

CONTINUOUS MURMUR

1. Heard in both systole and diastole.
2. Usually results from arteriovenous communication, usually from a patent ductus arteriosus.

PERICARDIAL FRICTION RUB

1. Leathery, scratchy, high-pitched, multiphasic extracardiac sound.
2. Cardiac phases of audible friction rub include ventricular systole, early ventricular diastole, and atrial systole.
3. Little radiation with pericardial friction rub; frequently best heard at the 3rd and 4th left sternal interspaces.
4. Etiologies include pericardial inflammation and insult.

BRUIT

1. Abnormal audible result of turbulent blood flowing through an artery, as in occlusive artery disease.
2. Auscultate with the bell of the stethoscope where arteries are closest to the surface (e.g., on the carotids).

THRILL

Vibrations that can be felt (on the precordium or AV shunt) as a result of turbulent blood flow.

B. BREATH SOUNDS

LOCATION OF BREATH SOUNDS

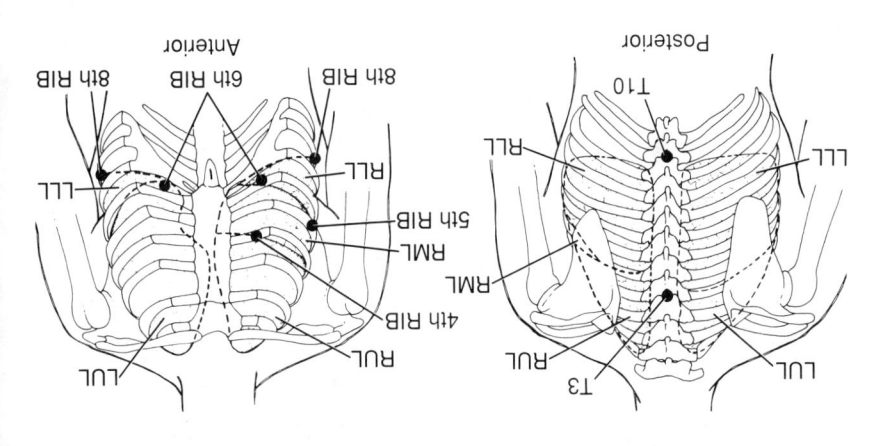

Figure 4.2

1. Upper and lower lobes are auscultated posteriorly.
2. Right middle lobe and both upper lobes are auscultated anteriorly.

NORMAL BREATH SOUNDS

1. Vesicular.
2. Bronchial.
3. Bronchovesicular.

VESICULAR SOUNDS

1. Heard over the periphery of the lung fields.
2. Low-pitched, rustling sound with no audible pause between inspiration and expiration.

BRONCHIAL SOUNDS
(Tracheal Sounds)

1. Normally only heard over the trachea.
2. Loud and high pitched.
3. Noticeable pause between inspiration and expiration.

BRONCHOVESICULAR SOUNDS

1. Heard over the major airways.
2. Characteristics are similar to combination of vesicular and bronchial sounds.

ABNORMAL BREATH SOUNDS

1. Bronchial breathing.
2. Euphony ("E to A" changes).
3. Whispered pectoriloquy.
4. Rales.
5. Rhonchi.
6. Wheezes.
7. Rhonchus.
8. Pleural friction rub.

BRONCHIAL BREATHING

1. Loud, high-pitched sounds heard over much of the lung field.
2. Results from pulmonary consolidation as seen in pneumonia or pleural effusion.

EUPHONY ("E TO A" CHANGES)

1. Sometimes heard with bronchial breathing.
2. Through the stethoscope, the patient saying "E" sounds like "A."

WHISPERED PECTORILOQUY

1. Patient's whispers sound much louder through the stethoscope.
2. Heard over areas of consolidation, pneumothorax, and pleural effusion when these areas communicate with a bronchus.

RALES

1. Fine to medium rales are produced in the small to medium airways, as at the bases.
2. Crackling sounds on inspiration.
3. Suspect left ventricular failure and pneumonia.

RHONCHI

1. Coarse rales.
2. Continuous bubbling, rattling sounds.
3. Suspect left ventricular failure and pneumonia.

WHEEZES

1. Airway narrowing.
2. High-pitched, whistle-like, musical sounds.
3. Heard during expiration.

RHONCHUS

1. Caused by retained secretions.
2. Wheeze-like sounds heard during both inspiration and expiration.

PLEURAL FRICTION RUB

1. A coarse, low-pitched, grating sound heard only during respiration.
2. Etiology is pleural fluid loss and inflammation that result in two pleural surfaces rubbing together.
3. Friction rub is loudest directly over the involved area.

SECTION 5

Lab Data

ARTERIAL BLOOD GASES

Normal Values

pH	7.35–7.45
pCO_2	35–45 mm Hg
pO_2	80–100 (room air) mm Hg
HCO_3	22–26 mmol/liter
O_2 saturation	97% (room air)

BLOOD CHEMISTRIES

(Normal values will vary among labs.)

Glucose	70–110 mg/100 ml (fasting)
Alkaline phosphate	30–85 units
Calcium	8.5–10.5 mg/100 ml
PO_4	2.5–4.5 mg/100 ml
Uric acid	2.5–8.0 mg/100 ml
Cholesterol	140–200 mg/100 ml
Total protein	6.0–8.0 mg/100 ml
Albumin	3.5–5.0 mg/100 ml

CARDIAC ENZYMES

1. CPK (creatinine phosphokinase)
2. LDH (lactic dehydrogenase)
3. SGOT (serum glutamic oxalacetic transaminase)

CPK

Normal = 6–30 units.

Elevates in 2–5 hours post MI.

Peaks during first 24 hours.

Peak = 5–15 times normal.

Returns to normal by 3rd day.

CPK-MB isoenzyme specific for MI.

LDH

Normal = 150–300 units.

Elevates 6–12 hours post MI.

Peaks in 48–72 hours.

Peak = 2–8 times normal.

Returns to normal in 5–6 days.

LDH_1 greater than LDH_2 is suggestive of MI.

Normally, LDH_2 is greater than LDH_1.

SGOT

Normal = 12–40 units.

Elevation occurs 6 hours post MI.

Peaks in 24–48 hours.

Peak = 2–15 times normal.

Returns to normal after 3-4 days.

ELECTROLYTES

(Normal values will vary among laboratories.)

Cl	95–105 mEq/liter
Na	135–145 mEq/liter
K	3.5–5.0 mEq/liter
CO_2	24–32 mEq/liter
BUN	6–17 mg/dl
Creatinine	male: 0.6–1.2 mg/dl
	female: 0.5–0.8 mg/dl

SECTION 6

Cardiac Drugs

AMIODARONE HCl
(Cordarone)

USES   Control ventricular and supraventricular dysrhythmias.

DOSAGE 1. 5-10 mg/kg i.v. is loading dose in adults (use central line).
2. Follow with 10 mg/kg i.v. for 3-5 days.
3. Oral maintenance dose is 200-400 mg/day.

ADVERSE 1. Bradycardia, hypotension, contractility, torsades de pointes, and other dysrhythmias.
2. Altered thyroid and liver functions.
3. Peripheral neuropathy, photosensitivity, corneal microdeposits.

4. Pulmonary fibrosis (incidence of 6–16% with 10% of these fatal).
5. Potentiates effect of warfarin and digoxin.
   Therapeutic level: 0.5–2.5 μg/ml

NOTE: All dosages are for adults unless otherwise indicated.

AMRINONE LACTATE
(Inocor Lactate Injection)

USES
1. Short-term management of congestive heart failure (CHF) and CHF symptoms (e.g., edema, dyspnea, orthopnea, fatigue).
2. Improve exercise tolerance in patients with CHF.
3. Short-term management of CHF patients who have not had adequate response to digitalis, diuretics, and/or vasodilators. Monitor usage closely because of amrinone's adverse reactions.

DOSAGE
1. Initially, 0.75-mg/kg bolus over 2–3 minutes.
2. Maintenance i.v. drip of 5 μg/kg/min to 10 μg/kg/min.

     3. An additional bolus of 0.75 mg/kg may be needed 30 minutes after the first bolus.

     4. Total daily dose should not exceed 10 mg/kg (however, use of up to 18 mg/kg has been reported).

ADVERSE   1. Thrombocytopenia (appears reversible), hepatotoxicity (with prolonged oral usage).

     2. Dysrhythmias, hypotension, chest pain.

     3. Nausea, vomiting, abdominal pain, anorexia.

NOTE: 1. Dilute in 1/2 normal saline solution (NS) or NS, and not with solutions containing dextrose.

ATENOLOL
(Tenormin)

USES Treat hypertension.

DOSAGE 1. 25–50 mg orally per day for initial 7–14 days.
2. May then increase to 200 mg/day.
3. Dosage may require adjustment in patients with impaired renal function.

ADVERSE 1. Hypotension, CHF, bradycardia, "masks diabetes mellitus."
2. Rash, fever, nausea, vomiting, diarrhea.
3. Lethargy, fatigue.
4. Caution in chronic obstructive pulmonary disease (COPD), concomitant use of Ca^{++} entry blockers.

ATROPINE SULFATE
(Atropine)

USES
1. Increase or restore heart rate.
2. Reduce degree of atrioventricular (AV) block.

DOSAGE
1. 0.3–0.5 mg intravenous push (IVP) every 5 minutes until 2.0 mg is given or the desired effect is reached.
2. Emergent endotracheal use: 0.5 mg/5 cc of NS.

ADVERSE
1. PVCs and V-tach.
2. Urinary retention, dry mouth, acute glaucoma, decreased bronchial secretions.
3. Mental confusion.

4. May increase myocardial infarct size (secondary to increased myocardial, oxygen consumption).

BRETYLIUM TOSYLATE
(Bretylol)

USES   Treat V-tach and V-fib that are refractory to xylocaine, quinidine, procainamide, and countershock.

DOSAGE 1. 5–10 mg/kg IVP for refractory V-fib.
2. 2.5–30 mg/kg every 4–6 hours intravenous piggyback (IVPB) over 10 minutes for V-tach or as continuous infusion at 1–2 mg/min.

ADVERSE 1. May potentiate digitalis-induced dysrhythmias.
2. May potentiate hypotensive effects of quinidine and propranolol.
3. Nausea and vomiting from rapid administration.
4. Confers increased sensitivity to catecholamines.

5. Avoid use in patients with increased intracranial pressures.
   Therapeutic level: 0.5–1.5 mg/ml

CALCIUM

USES 1. In cardiac arrest, to increase myocardial tone and contractions when patient is hypocalcemic and hyperkalemic secondary to calcium blocker toxicity.
2. Make V-fib movements coarser.

DOSAGE 1. Adults: calcium chloride 10% solution, 3–5 cc IVP over 3 minutes.
2. Children: calcium gluconate 10% solution 10 cc IVPB.

ADVERSE 1. Cardiac arrest with rapid infusion.
2. Potentiates digitalis toxicity.
3. Hypercalcemia.

NOTE: Never mix with sodium bicarbonate.

CAPTOPRIL
(Capoten)

USES Treat severe hypertension, refractory CHF (use smaller doses starting at 6.25 mg every 8 hours).

DOSAGE 1. Initial dosage 25 mg TID.
2. If hypertension not satisfactory after 1-2 weeks, slowly titrate dosage up to maximum dosage of 450 mg TID.

ADVERSE 1. Tachycardia, hypotension, CHF, angina, pericarditis.
2. Renal failure, hyperkalemia, anorexia, skin rash, fever, neutropenia, proteinuria.

3. Vertigo, syncope.
4. Metallic taste sense.

NOTE: If lower dosages of captopril do not control hypertension, it may be necessary to add a diuretic.

CLONIDINE HCl
(Catapres)

USES   Treat hypertension (essential, renal, malignant).

DOSAGE 1. Starting dose: 0.1 mg BID.
2. May increase dosage to 0.2 mg daily p.o. gradually.
3. Maximum daily dosage is 2.4 mg in divided doses.

ADVERSE 1. Bradycardia; hypotension, especially orthostatic hypotension.
2. Vertigo, drowsiness, headache, nervousness.
3. Urinary retention, constipation, impotence.
4. Caution in chronic renal failure, recent MI, severe coronary insufficiency.
5. Rebound hypertension upon abrupt discontinuation.

DIAZEPAM
(Valium)

USES Create amnesia for elective cardioversion.

DOSAGE 0.1–0.2 mg/min IVP until dose of 5–15 mg is reached.

ADVERSE
1. Hypotension, bradycardia, tachycardia.
2. Increased cough reflex, laryngospasm, apnea.
3. Slurred speech, phlebitis, venous thrombosis.
4. Cardiac arrest.

Therapeutic level: 0.1–2.2 μg/ml

DIGOXIN
(Lanoxin)

USES 1. Treat supraventricular dysrhythmias (use cautiously in Wolff-Parkinson-White syndrome).
2. Treat CHF (increases cardiac output).

DOSAGE 1. Loading dose: 0.5–1.0 mg IVP in divided doses.
2. Maintenance dose: 0.125–0.5 mg/day.

ADVERSE 1. Almost any dysrhythmia.
2. Neurologic and gastrointestinal disturbances.

3. Gynecomastia, skin rash.
4. AV block.
   Therapeutic level: 0.6–2.0 ng/ml (for CHF); may exceed 2.0 ng/ml for atrial fibrillation as tolerated.

DILTIAZEM
(Cardizem)

USES
1. Manage Prinzmetal's (vasospastic or variant) angina.
2. Manage stable angina.

DOSAGE
1. Initial dose: 30 mg orally QID.
2. Titrate up to 360 mg daily in divided doses.

ADVERSE
1. Hypotension, bradycardia, dysrhythmias, conduction anomalies, edema.
2. Vertigo, confusion, drowsiness, headache, nervousness.

3. Nausea, vomiting, diarrhea; transient elevation of liver function tests; photosensitivity.

NOTE: Use cautiously with other beta blockers because of potential for prolonged cardiac conduction time.

DIPYRIDAMOLE
(Persantine)

USES
1. Increase coronary blood flow without significant alteration of systemic blood pressure.
2. Long-term treatment of angina pain.
3. Post myocardial infarction in combination with acetylsalicylic acid (aspirin) for antiplatelet effect.

DOSAGE
50-75 mg p.o. TID before meals.

ADVERSE
1. Headache, vertigo.
2. Syncope, flushing, skin rash.
3. Nausea.

DISOPYRAMIDE
(Norpace)

USES
1. Treat PVCs.
2. Prevent V-tach.

DOSAGE
1. Loading dose: 300 mg p.o.
2. 50–300 mg p.o. every 6–8 hours.

ADVERSE
1. Urinary hesitancy and retention.
2. Dryness of eyes, nose, mouth, throat.
3. Nausea, constipation, bloating, gas pain.
4. Vertigo, fatigue, headache, malaise, syncope, shortness of breath, hypotension.
5. Myocardial depression, hypotension, torsades de pointes, electromechanical dissociation.

6. Use with caution in combination with beta blockers, digitalis, and other class I antiarrhythmics.
Therapeutic level: 2–8 μg/ml.

DOBUTAMINE HCl
(Dobutrex)

USES 1. Treat cardiogenic shock (inotropic effect).
2. Short-term treatment of decompensation.

DOSAGE 1. Commonly, 2.5–10 μg/kg/min i.v. drip.
2. Occasionally, doses to 40 μg/kg/min.

ADVERSE 1. Increased heart rate, PVCs, increased systolic blood pressure.
2. Increased AV conduction (for patients with atrial fibrillation, give digitalis before starting Dobutrex).
3. Nausea, headache, dyspnea, angina, palpitations.
4. Inactivated by sodium bicarbonate, heparin.

DOPAMINE HCl
(Intropin)

USES
1. Treatment of choice for cardiogenic shock.
2. Treat decompensation, other shock.
3. Increase renal perfusion.

DOSAGE
1. Titrate 2–50 μg/kg/min for cardiogenic shock.
2. Titratae 2–5 μg/kg/min for renal perfusion.

ADVERSE
1. Dysrhythmias.
2. Nausea, vomiting, dyspnea, headache.
3. Hypertension, vasoconstriction.
4. Extravasation → sloughing.

NOTE: pH incompatibility with sodium bicarbonate. Do not mix dopamine
with $NaCHO_3$.

EDROPHONIUM CHLORIDE
(Tensilon)

USES   Treat atrial tachycardia.

DOSAGE   Titrate 2–10 mg IVP until tachycardia breaks; maximum: 40 mg.

ADVERSE 1. Bradycardia, cardiac standstill, hypotension.
2. Convulsions, weakness.
3. Increased bronchial secretions, respiratory muscle paralysis, larynogospasm.
4. Contains sodium sulfite, i.e., can cause anaphylaxis.

EPINEPHRINE HCl
(Adrenalin)

USES
1. Initiate cardiac rhythm in arrest.
2. Reduce degree of heart block (largely supplanted by pacemakers).
3. Increase blood pressure (less potent vasoconstrictor than norepinephrine).

DOSAGE
1. 5 ml of 1:10,000 solution every 5 minutes.
2. 7.5–15 μg/kg every 5 minutes; maximum: 5–15 mg.
3. Emergent endotracheal route: 15–30 μg/kg.
4. 0.5 ml of 1:1,000 solution every 5 minutes (not seen often in adult setting); continuous infusion: 1–4 μg/min.

ADVERSE 1. Ventricular dysrhythmias.
2. Angina, headache, tremor.
3. Reduced urinary output.
4. Fear, anxiety.

ERYTHRITYL TETRANITRATE
(Cardilate)

USES   Prevent and treat recurrent angina.

DOSAGE   1. 5 mg sublingually TID.
2. 10 mg (chewable tablets) before meals TID.
3. Increase dose as needed in 48–72 hours; maximum: 100 mg/day.

ADVERSE   1. Tachycardia, orthostatic hypotension, palpitations, syncope.
2. Headache (sometimes throbbing), vertigo, weakness.
3. Nausea, vomiting.

HYDRALAZINE HCl
(Apresoline)

USES 1. Treat essential hypertension.

2. Reduce afterload in CHF and cardiogenic shock.

DOSAGE 1. Intravenous: 10–40 mg IVPB or slow IVP initially; then repeat every 4–6 hours PRN; change to oral administration when practical.

2. Intramuscular: 20–40 mg every 4–6 hours or repeat as necessary.

3. Orally: generally 50-200 mg daily in divided doses; some patients require up to 400 mg daily total in divided doses.

ADVERSE 1. Tachycardia, orthostatic hypotension, angina, palpitations, dysrhythmias.
2. Headache, vertigo, peripheral neuritis.
3. Nausea, vomiting, diarrhea, anorexia.
4. Lupus-like syndrome, rash, sodium retention, weight gain.

ISOPROTERENOL HCl
(Isuprel)

USES
1. Increase pacemaker automaticity and AV conduction.
2. Treat cardiogenic shock.
3. Bronchodilation.

DOSAGE
1. I.V.: titrate 0.5–10 μg/min.
2. IC: 0.02 mg direct push over 1-2 minutes.

ADVERSE
1. SVT, PVCs, V-tach, V-fib, death.
2. Hypotension from vasodilation, decreased coronary perfusion pressure.
3. Headache, flushing, angina, nausea, tremor, vertigo, weakness, sweating.

ISOSORBIDE DINITRATE
(Sorbitrate, Isordil)

USES
1. Prophylaxis and treatment of acute (sublingual, chewable) and chronic (oral) angina.
2. Treat chronic ischemic heart disease.
3. Used with other vasodilator drugs to treat chronic CHF.

DOSAGE
1. Sublingual: 2.5–10 mg; may repeat in 2–3 hours PRN for acute angina, and routinely 4–6 hours for prophylaxis.
2. Chewable: 5–10 mg; may repeat in 2-3 hours for acute angina.
3. Oral: 5–40 mg every 6–8 hours for prophylaxis.

ADVERSE 1. Hypotension (especially orthostatic hypotension), tachycardia, palpitations, syncope.
2. Headache, vertigo, weakness, flushing.
3. Nausea, vomiting, sublingual tingling/burning (confirms drug action).
4. In patients with outlet obstruction, that is, valvular stenosis or idiopathic hypertrophic subaortic stenosis, use caution; observe for decreased cardiac output, pulmonary edema.

NOTE: 1. Use test dose to determine that symptomatic hypotension will not result from this drug.
2. Use the smallest effective dosage.
3. Antagonizes action of norepinephrine.

LABETALOL HCl
(Normodyne, Trandate)

USES Treat hypertension.

DOSAGE
1. Initial dose: start with 100 mg orally BID.
2. May increase to 200 mg orally BID after 2–3 days, and further increase every 2–3 days until effective dosage is reached.
3. Usual maintenance dose: between 200 mg and 400 mg BID.
4. Hypertensive emergency: 20–60 mg IVP followed by 2-mg/min infusion.

ADVERSE
1. Orthostatic hypotension, vertigo.
2. Headache, weakness, impotence.

3. Nausea, vomiting, urinary retention.
4. Rash, hypoglycemia, vivid dreams.
5. Ventricular dysrhythmias.

LIDOCAINE HCl
(Xylocaine)

USES
1. Suppress ventricular ectopy associated with acute MI.
2. Treat ventricular dysrhythmias associated with cardiac surgery and digitalis toxicity.

DOSAGE
1. 0.5–1 mg/kg slow IVP over 2–3 minutes; then 1–4 mg/min i.v. infusion after loading dose, followed by 0.5 mg/kg "2nd bolus" at 10 minutes after loading bolus.
2. Emergent endotrachael dose: 1 mg/kg in 10–25 ml of H_2O or NS.

ADVERSE 1. CNS depression, agitation, convulsions, coma, death.
2. Hypotension, tremor (usually first sign of toxicity), circulatory collapse.
Therapeutic level: 1.2–6 μg/ml

METARAMINOL BITARTRATE
(Aramine)

USES 1. Treat hypotension.
2. Terminate supraventricular dysrhythmias.

DOSAGE 1. 100 mg in 250 ml of solution; titrate to desired effect; start at 5 µg/min.
2. Emergent i.v. dose 5 mg IVP.
3. 2–10 mg i.m. every 10 minutes to prevent cumulative effect.

ADVERSE 1. Reflex bradycardia.
2. Ventricular dysrhythmias.
3. Tissue sloughing from s.c. injections.

METHOXAMINE HCl
(Vasoxyl)

USES
1. Treat PAT.
2. Reverse excessive hypotension caused by ganglion-blocking agents.
3. Treat shock with low peripheral resistance.

DOSAGE
1. 0.1 mg/kg slow i.v. injection.
2. For PAT, average dose is 10 mg slow IVP; infusion 5 μg/min to start.
3. Repeat not sooner than 15 minutes with 10–15 mg i.m. if needed.

ADVERSE
1. Hypovolemia, decreased plasma volume.
2. Headache, pilomotor stimulation, projectile emesis.

3. Bradycardia, exacerbation of CHF (2nd degree hypertension), sinus arrest.
4. Severe hypertensive crisis when used concomitantly with beta blockers, tricyclic antidepressants, monoamine oxidase inhibitors, reserpine, guanethidine.

METHYLDOPA
(Aldomet)

USES   Treat chronic hypertension.

DOSAGE 1. Initial dose: 250 mg orally 2–3 times a day.
2. May increase after 48 hours and every 48 hours thereafter until maintenance level is reached.
3. Maintenance dose: usually 500–2000 mg daily in divided doses.

ADVERSE 1. Bradycardia, orthostatic hypotension, increased angina, carditis.
2. Drowsiness, reversible hemolytic anemia, weakness, vertigo, decreased mentation.

3. Psychic dysfunctions, headache, diarrhea, hepatic necrosis, rash, fever.
4. Potentiation of pressor effects of sympathomimetics.

NOTE: An i.v. form is available for use in hospitals.

METOPROLOL TARTRATE
(Lopressor)

USES Treat hypertension, post MI prophylaxis (reduce infarct size).

DOSAGE 1. Intravenous bolus dose 5 mg IVP every 2 minutes × 3 doses, then 50 mg p.o. every 6 hours for 48 hours, then 100 mg p.o. BID.
2. Initial dose: 50–100 mg/day orally in single or divided dose.
3. Increase to 200–400 mg daily in divided dose.

ADVERSE 1. Hypotension, bradycardia, CHF, peripheral vascular disease.

2. Fatigue, lethargy, rash, fever, "masks diabetes mellitus."
3. Nausea, vomiting.

MEXILETINE HCl
(Mexitil)

USES Treat refractory ventricular dysrhythmias, e.g., PVC, V-tach.

DOSAGE 1. Intravenous bolus of 200–250 mg over 3–5 minutes.
2. Follow with infusion of 0.5–1.5 mg/min.
3. Oral dose for maintenance: 150–400 mg p.o. every 6–8 hours.

ADVERSE 1. Bradycardia, hypotension, widened QRS complex.
2. Tremor, vertigo, CNS symptoms, visual disturbances.

3. Nausea, vomiting, rash.
Therapeutic level: 0.5–2 μg/ml.

NOTE: Mexiletine interacts with phenytoin, phenobarbital, and rifampin, resulting in lowered mexiletine levels. Monitor carefully when these drugs are used.

MORPHINE

USES 1. Relieve severe pain.
2. Treat pulmonary edema.

DOSAGE Titrate 2–10 mg slow (over 5 minutes) IVP or IVPB every 1–3 hours.

ADVERSE 1. Hypotension, drowsiness, coma, nausea, vomiting, constipation, urinary retention.
2. Respiratory arrest, apnea.
Therapeutic level: 0.1–0.5 μg/ml

NOTE: Contraindicated post biliary surgery or gut reanastomosis; increases action of some anticoagulants (Coumarin); cautious concomitant use of monoamine oxidase inhibitors.

NADOLOL
(Corgard)

USES Treat angina, hypertension.

DOSAGE 1. Initial dose: 40 mg orally single daily dose.
2. Increase dose 40–80 mg until desired result is reached; maximum: 240 mg/day.

ADVERSE 1. Hypotension, bradycardia, CHF, peripheral vascular disease.
2. Lethargy and fatigue, rash, fever.
3. Nausea, vomiting, diarrhea, increased airway resistance.
4. Masks diabetes mellitus.

NALOXONE HCl
(Narcan)

USES   Treat narcotic-induced depression, especially respiratory.

DOSAGE 1. 0.4 mg (1 ml) i.v., i.m., or s.c.
2. Repeat above dosage at 2- to 3-minute intervals for up to 5 doses (2 mg).

ADVERSE 1. Adverse effects are related to rate of reversal of analgesia or intoxication.
2. Nausea, vomiting, hypertension, sweating.

NOTE: Do not mix with alkaline solutions, e.g., sodium bicarbonate.

NITROGLYCERIN

USES
1. Prophylaxis and treatment of angina, both acute and chronic (oral, sublingual, topical).
2. Produce controlled hypotension during surgery (i.v.).
3. Treat CHF associated with MI and ischemic episodes (preload reduction) i.v.

DOSAGE
1. Topical: 2% ointment; start with one-half inch and increase until desired effect is reached; usual dose is 1–2 inches TID.
2. Sublingual: 0.2–0.6 mg for acute angina; may repeat every 5 minutes for 3 doses.
3. Oral: 1 sustained-release capsule every 8-12 hours.

4. Intravenous: start at 5 μg/min; titrate up every 3–5 minutes until relief of chest pain or hypotension is achieved.

ADVERSE 1. Hypotension (especially orthostatic), flushing, tachycardia, syncope.
2. Headache, vertigo, weakness.
3. Nausea, vomiting.

NITROPRUSSIDE SODIUM
(Nipride)

USES
1. Immediate treatment of hypertensive crisis.
2. Produce controlled hypotension during surgery to minimize blood loss.
3. Treat cardiogenic shock (preload and afterload reduction).

DOSAGE   Titrate (not to exceed 10 μg/kg/min).

ADVERSE
1. Sudden, severe hypotension.
2. Chest and abdominal pain.
3. Neurologic disturbances.
4. Nausea, vomiting.
5. Cyanide toxicity.

NOREPINEPHRINE
(Levophed)

USES 1. Treat cardiogenic shock.
2. Treat other severe forms of hypotension.

DOSAGE 1. 1–2 μg/min i.v.
2. Titrate solution for desired effect (adequate cardiac output).

ADVERSE 1. Severe hypertension.
2. Tissue sloughing from infiltration (use a central line if one is available); treat extravasation by infiltrating with phentolamine.
3. Many and varied dysrhythmias.
4. Anxiety, headache.

PHENTOLAMINE HCl
(Regitine)

USES 1. Vasodilation to inhibit hypertension due to high levels of epinephrine and norepinephrine.
2. Reduce tissue sloughing caused by Levophed infiltration.
3. Aid in diagnosis of pheochromocytoma.

DOSAGE 1. 5–15 mg 4–6 times a day i.v. for vasodilation.
2. 10 mg in 10 ml of 5% dextrose in water injection (D_5W) or normal saline s.c. to infiltrated area within 12 hours of extravasation.

ADVERSE 1. Tachycardia, orthostatic hypotension, acute MI, cerebrovascular accident, cerebrovascular spasm.
2. Nausea, vomiting, diarrhea.
3. Weakness, vertigo, flushing.

PHENYLEPHRINE HCl
(Neo-Synephrine)

USES
1. Reverse hypotension.
2. Treat shock from decreased peripheral resistance.
3. Treat PAT.

DOSAGE
1. 0.1–0.5 mg i.v. push; repeat dose not sooner than 10–15 minutes.
2. 10 mg in 500 ml of D_5W = 1:50,000 continuous infusion 100–180 µg/min, then 40–60 µg/min when blood pressure responds.
3. 5–10 mg s.c. or i.m.

ADVERSE 1. Tachycardia, hypertension, sweating, palpitations.
2. Use with caution in cases of hypertension, slow heart rate, block, myocardial disease.

PHENYTOIN SODIUM
(Dilantin)

USES 1. Treat digitalis-induced dysrhythmias, such as atrial tachycardia with block, PVCs.
2. Depress pacemaker activity.

DOSAGE 50–100 mg i.v. over 5–10 minutes (maximum rate: 50 mg/min) until dysrhythmia is corrected (maximum dose: 15 mg/kg).

ADVERSE 1. Significant hypotension after rapid i.v. infusion.
2. Pain and phlebitis, ataxia, vertigo, seizures.
3. Nausea, vomiting.
4. Decreases warfarin action by increasing clearance of warfarin.

Therapeutic level: 10–20 μg/ml as anticonvulsant, but for digitalis toxicity much higher levels may be needed.

NOTE: Will precipitate in D$_5$W; give with normal saline.

PINDOLOL
(Visken)

USES   Treat hypertension.

DOSAGE   1. Initial dose: 5–10 mg BID orally.
2. May increase by 10 mg/day every 48-72 hours.
3. Maximum dose: 60 mg/day in divided doses.

ADVERSE 1. Bradycardia, tachycardia, CHF, hypotension, peripheral vascular disease.
2. Vertigo, insomnia, other CNS symptoms.
3. Nausea, vomiting, visual disturbances, rash, masks diabetes mellitus.

POTASSIUM CHLORIDE

USES
1. Treat and prevent ventricular dysrhythmias, especially those associated with digitalis toxicity.
2. Treat hypokalemia.
3. Treat digitalis toxicity if there are no conduction defects.

DOSAGE
1. Intravenous: 5–15 mEq/50 ml of D_5W or normal saline infused over 1 hour.
2. Maintenance: 20–80 mEq daily p.o.; other oral dosage as indicated by lab results.

ADVERSE
1. Bradycardia, depression of pacemaker cells, slowing of conduction to the point of heart block.
2. EKG changes.

3. Vein irritation.
4. Cardiac arrest.
5. Caution in renal insufficiency.

PRAZOSIN HCl
(Minipress)

USES
1. Treat mild to moderate hypertension.
2. Decrease afterload in refractory CHF.

DOSAGE
1. Initial dose: 1 mg p.o. at bedtime or with patient on bed rest to minimize risk of initial dose syncope, falling, injury.
2. Maintenance dose: usually between 3 and 20 mg daily.

ADVERSE
1. Hypotension (especially orthostatic), tachycardia, palpitations, syncope.

2. Vertigo, headache, drowsiness.
3. Blurred vision, vomiting, diarrhea, abdominal cramping.

NOTE: If used with other antihypertensives or diuretics, anticipate reducing prazosin dosage.

PROCAINAMIDE HCl
(Pronestyl, Procan SR)

USES 1. Treat PVCs refractory to lidocaine.
2. Treat virtually all dysrhythmias.

DOSAGE 1. Intravenous loading dose: usually 100 mg slow IVP (maximum rate: 20 mg/min); repeat every 5 minutes until dysrhythmias are controlled, then 2–6 mg/min i.v. (loading dose of 1000–1250 mg over 60–90 minutes).
2. Oral loading dose: 1000 mg.
3. Maintenance dose: 50 mg/kg/day in divided doses.
4. Sustained-release oral tablets maintenance dose: 500–1000 mg every 6 hours.

ADVERSE
1. Hypotension, cardiovascular collapse, convulsions, coronary insufficiency, AV block, PVCs, 1:1 conduction of atrial flutter, torsades de pointes.
2. Lupus syndrome after prolonged use.
3. CNS disturbances.
4. Hematologic dyscrasias: neutropenia, pancytopenia, thrombocytopenia.
   Therapeutic level for procainamide: 4–8 μg/ml; for *N*-acetyl-procainamide (active metabolite): 10–15 μg/ml.

PROPRANOLOL HCl
(Inderal)

USES 1. Control ventricular response to atrial fibrillation, atrial flutter, and atrial tachycardia.
2. Suppress ectopic discharge and PAT.
3. Treat angina.
4. Acute MI infarct size reduction.
5. Chronic treatment of hypertension.

DOSAGE 1. Intravenous: 0.5–1.0 mg every 1–3 minutes slow IVP (maximum: 0.1 mg/kg).
2. Oral: 10–80 mg every 6–8 hours.

ADVERSE 1. Hypotension, bradycardia, CHF.
2. CNS disturbances.

3. Nausea, vomiting, diarrhea, rash, masks diabetes mellitus.
4. Increased airway resistance.
   Therapeutic level: 0.05–0.1 μg/ml.

NOTE: 1. Myocardial depressant: do not give where AV block or CHF exists.
    2. Contraindicated also with asthma, COPD, or recent verapamil or Dilantin use.

QUINIDINE
(GLUCONATE AND SULFATE)
(Quinaglute and Quinidine)

USES 1. Treat virtually all dysrhythmias (i.v. for rapid control).
2. Decrease strength of myocardial contraction.
3. Reduce conduction velocity in the myocardium.

DOSAGE 1. Quinaglute: usual maintenance dose is 324–648 mg every 6–8 hours.
2. Quinidine: usual maintenance dose between 200 and 600 mg every 3–4 hours (6 mg/kg every 4–6 hours).

ADVERSE 1. Hypotension, respiratory depression, convulsions, death.

2. Increased CHF, SA and AV block, asystole.
3. Idioventricular rhythms, V-fib, torsades de pointes (especially when potassium is decreased).
4. Thrombocytopenia.
5. Twofold elevation of digitalis levels when quinidine is added.

Therapeutic level: 2–6 μg/ml

NOTE: Patient should be given digitals before starting quinidine to avoid increasing AV conduction (AV conduction velocity is initially increased with quinidine, then slows).

SODIUM BICARBONATE

USES   Treat acidosis (lactic acidosis).

DOSAGE 1. In cardiac arrest: 1 mEq/kg initially (although use is now seriously questioned).
2. One-half initial dose every 10 minutes PRN.

ADVERSE 1. Metabolic alkalosis from excess $NaHCO_3$ (alkalemia, hyperosmolality, sodium overload).
2. Large amounts may worsen CHF.
3. Inactivates catecholamines.

TIMOLOL MALEATE
(Blocadren)

USES Treat hypertension, post MI prophylaxis (reduce infarct size).

DOSAGE 1. Initial dose: 10 mg p.o. BID.
2. Usual maintenance dose: 10–30 mg BID.
3. Maximum daily dosage: 60 mg.

ADVERSE 1. Hypotension, bradycardia, CHF, masks diabetes mellitus.
2. Weakness, lethargy, fatigue.
3. Nausea, vomiting, diarrhea, rash.
4. Peripheral vascular disease, increased airway resistance.

VERAPAMIL HCl
(Calan, Isoptin)

USES
1. Manage stable and chronic angina.
2. Manage Prinzmetal's or variant (vasospastic) angina.
3. Convert SVT if carotid massage is unsuccessful (use with caution if recent beta-blocker use, WPW syndrome, or CHF).

DOSAGE
1. Intravenous: 0.075–0.15 mg/kg slow IVP over two minutes or IVPB (with blood pressure and EKG monitoring); repeat in 10–15 minutes PRN (SVT); maximum 15 mg/30 min.
2. Oral: 80 mg 3–4 times a day; maintenance dose may be as high as 480 mg/day.

ADVERSE 1. Bradycardia, transient hypotension, CHF, AV block, asystole.
2. Vertigo, headache, fatigue.
3. Nausea, constipation, elevated liver function tests.
4. Use with caution in patients who have just received i.v. propranolol or a recent high dose of oral beta blockers.

Therapeutic level: 0.08–0.3 μg/ml

SECTION 7

Terminology

ABERRANT VENTRICULAR CONDUCTION

1. Transient conduction that is partially blocked, resulting in a wide, bizarre, abnormal QRS.
2. Etiologies include premature atrial contractions, rapid rates, and changes in cycle length. The His-Purkinje system has not completed repolarization and impulses cannot conduct normally.

ADRENERGIC DRUG EFFECTS

1. Alpha = peripheral vasoconstriction.
2. Beta$_1$ = increased heart rate and contractile force.
3. Beta$_2$ = visceral vasodilation, especially pulmonic vascular bed.

AFTERLOAD

1. Resistance the left ventricle must work against to pump blood into the systemic circulation.
2. As afterload increases, less volume is ejected, which leads to decreased stroke volume.
3. Left and right ventricular afterload can be approximated clinically by measuring systemic and pulmonary pressures.

ALPHA-BETA MIMETIC

1. Levophed, Adrenalin, Aramine.
2. Alpha mimetic = peripheral vasoconstriction with increase in blood pressure.
3. Beta mimetic = positive inotropic and chronotropic action.

ALPHA LYTIC

1. Regitine, Dibenzyline.
2. Produce reduced arterial and venous constriction that is caused by alpha-mimetic drugs.
3. Acts like beta receptor stimulation of peripheral blood vessels.

BETA LYTIC

1. Inderal.
2. Blocks inotropic and chronotropic actions of beta-receptor stimulation, decreases cardiac output, possibly increases arterial resistance.

BETA MIMETIC

1. Isuprel, Wyamine.
2. Results in increased cardiac output, decreased peripheral vascular resistance, decreased venous pooling, increased blood return to the heart, and positive inotropic and chronotropic action.

CHEYNE-STOKES RESPIRATIONS

1. Dysrhythmic breathing that varies from slow and shallow to fast and deep.
2. Seen in primary CNS disturbances and severe CHF.

CHRONOTROPIC

1. Refers to heart rate.
2. Positive chronotropic = increased rate.
3. Negative chronotropic = decreased rate.

DROMOTROPIC

1. Refers to conduction velocity.
2. Positive dromotropic = increased conduction.
3. Negative dromotropic = decreased conduction.

INOTROPIC

1. Refers to myocardial contractility.
2. Positive inotropic = strengthened contraction.
3. Negative inotropic = weakened contraction.

INOTROPIC DRUGS: NEGATIVE

1. Beta-blocking agents (Inderal).
2. Anesthesia.
3. Severe hypoxia.
4. Acidosis.

INOTROPIC DRUGS: POSITIVE

1. Digitalis.
2. Calcium.
3. Beta-adrenergic drugs (Isuprel, Levophed, Adrenalin).
4. Sympathetic nervous system stimulation.
5. Mild hypoxia.

KUSSMAUL RESPIRATIONS

Deep, gasping respirations seen in severe acidosis.

PRELOAD

1. The length to which myocardial fibers are stretched at the end of diastole (filling pressure).
2. As preload increases, the tension of the myocardial muscle increases, resulting in increased force of contraction and increased stroke volume (to a point).
3. Left ventricular preload is measured by the pulmonary artery wedge pressure.
4. Right ventricular preload is measured by the central venous pressure.

PRESSOR EFFECT

Increases blood pressure by increasing peripheral vasoconstriction.

REFRACTORY PERIOD

Period of myocardial relaxation during which excitability is depressed. If stimulated, the heart will respond but a stronger stimulus is required and response is less.

STOKES-ADAMS SYNDROME

1. Sudden attacks of weakness, syncope, sweating, and sometimes convulsions.
2. Caused by decreased cerebral perfusion.

SYMPATHOMIMETIC DRUGS
(Catecholamines)

1. Epinephrine, norepinephrine, dopamine, dobutamine, Isuprel.
2. Cause systemic arterial vasoconstriction, positive inotropic and positive chronotropic effects, and increased pulmonary circulation (dobutamine and Isuprel do not cause vasoconstriction).

VASOACTIVE DRUGS

1. Drugs that increase rate and volume increase systolic pressure.
2. Drugs that decrease rate and cause vasoconstriction affect diastolic pressure.

BIBLIOGRAPHY

Andreoli V, Zipes D, Wallace A, Kinney M, Fowkes V. *Comprehensive Cardiac Care*, ed 6. St. Louis, Mosby, 1987.

Conover M. *Understanding Electrocardiography*, ed 4. St. Louis, Mosby, 1984.

Marriott H. *Practical Electrocardiography*, ed 7. Baltimore, Williams & Wilkins, 1983.

Marriott H. *EKG/PDQ*. Baltimore, Williams & Wilkins, 1987.

Pechan M. *Coronary Care Modules*. Baltimore, Williams & Wilkins, 1987.

Purcell J. Pacemaker primer. *Am J Nurs* 85: 553–567, 1985.

Springhouse Corporation. *Nursing 87 Drug Handbook*. Springhouse, PA, Springhouse Corporation, 1987.